Dear
Happy writing!

THE
HEALTHY
WRITER

REDUCE YOUR PAIN, IMPROVE YOUR HEALTH, AND BUILD A WRITING CAREER FOR THE LONG-TERM

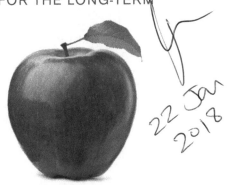

22 Jan
2018

Joanna Penn &
Dr Euan Lawson

Contents

Joanna's dedication:

For Jonathan, who taught me to breathe.

Euan's dedication:

For Sophie, Archie, Imogen and Summer.

Introduction

"We all have cracks. We just hide them from each other."

Ruby Wax, Sane New World

Writing is part of who we are, it's how we make sense of the world and how we connect with others through the page.

For some it's therapy, for others, it's income, but for all of us who call ourselves writers, it's an integral part of our lives. We cannot give up writing no matter what the cost.

But we are not just brains that pour words onto a page or a screen. We have a physical body that needs looking after if we are to make it through a long and happy life creating and writing and living life to the full.

The unfortunate truth is that writing can be an unhealthy way to spend your time and many writers end up with chronic physical pain issues and/or mental health problems along the way. Let's face it, hunching over for hours every day, eyes fixed on a bright screen, hands bashing away at a keyboard or scribbling on a page can result in conditions that hinder a full life.

But it doesn't have to be like this. You *can* be a healthy writer, and this book will show you the way.

I'm Joanna Penn, New York Times and USA Today best-selling thriller author (under J.F.Penn), non-fiction writer, podcaster and international speaker. I make my living from my writing and most of my days are spent creating words on the page for books, blog posts, emails or social media. I've suffered from many of the issues writers face – back pain, headaches and eye strain, repetitive strain injury, weight gain, stress and burnout – and I've spent the last five years trying to reduce my pain in order to have a happier, healthier writing life. I'll share my personal journey with you as well as what has worked for me.

My co-author is Euan Lawson, a British medical doctor, who brings the expertise and scientific point of view to the book as well as thoughts from his own experiences.

Together, we want to help writers reduce their pain and live a healthier life so we can all write for the long term. We hope that our combined approach will give a balanced view of what a healthy writer can be. The different chapters each give an indication who is writing, although sometimes we have merged together within one chapter. All the medical studies and references discussed are in Appendix 2.

Disclaimer: Although Euan is a doctor, he is not *your* doctor and this book is not medical advice. It contains thoughts, suggestions and information that we hope will help you, but please seek appropriate medical advice for your situation.

There is a risk that any book about health can get preachy, but this is a not a book about denial. It is not necessary to live a life that would make a monk weep. We are not aspirational ascetics, denying the flesh for the greater holiness of the written word. This is not an exhaustive book covering everything possible, but we hope it will help you feel less alone in your journey toward wellness.

It is about empowerment. It is about sustainability. It is about making change that will help you become a healthy writer for the long term.

How we decided what to include in the book

In a survey I ran on TheCreativePenn.com in August 2017, over 1100 writers answered questions that helped us put together the topics to focus on. The most common health issues reported were sedentary behavior/sitting too much, stress, back pain, weight gain, anxiety and sleep problems. Others reported headaches, eye strain, loneliness and depression, digestive issues, and Repetitive Strain Injury. There are quotes throughout from writers who agreed to share their problems and tips openly.

Thanks to everyone who responded and we hope that this book helps you with some of these issues and make your writing a sustainable career for the long-term.

We have much in common, but we are also individuals

People are infinitely variable and your experience of a medical problem is likely to be substantially different from another person's, even with the same diagnosis. It's part of the medical profession's role to sift and sort people, putting them into various boxes, adding labels to ease the process of finding the best possible ways to help. That's the science of medicine. The art has always been in recognizing that there are limitations to that when managing people.

You need to get to know your body and your mind over time. How you respond will be different to the next person, so you need to treat this health journey as a lifetime adventure, just as the writing life can continue until we breathe no more.

We all have layers of history written into our bodies – habits we've acquired, patterns of behavior and thinking that we repeat, and these can result in pain that must be peeled back, layer by layer, over time. You might find that you change one thing and then discover more issues underneath. This process is entirely normal, as you'll find with Joanna's personal journey to a pain-free back or Euan's shift from fat to fit later on.

So, why did you pick up this book?

Whatever comes to mind first is the place to start, but hopefully, you will also find more inside these pages that will help you as the layers drop away.

We can show you some directions to consider, but you will need to find your own way to a healthy creative life as a writer. We hope this book highlights some pitfalls and gives some pointers.

How to use this book

Part 1 outlines the most common health issues that writers face and offers some actions for how you can remedy the situation. Not all problems are applicable to everyone, so we hope that you will dip in and out of this section for anything that might help you over time.

Part 2 looks at ways you can reduce pain, build resilience into your life and actively move toward being a healthy writer. This section also gives you ideas and tips for improving your health even further and enjoying being active. Euan is a runner and Joanna has started walking ultra-marathons and we both share ideas on how to incorporate more activity into your writing life.

Note: We are both in the UK but our readers are international and we recognize that health care options and associated costs are different by country, so please weigh up any advice against your situation.

We don't cover the topic of disability in any significant detail, either physical or severe mental illness. If you have specific medical conditions, then you should take advice from your doctor before embarking on any new or exotic treatments.

"To keep the body in good health is a duty ... otherwise we shall not be able to keep our mind strong and clear."

Buddha

* * *

Please note: This book contains some affiliate links to products/services we recommend and use ourselves.

7 reasons why writing is great for your health

We are writers and many of us become grumpy if we go too long without writing. It is an intrinsic part of our lives. Some of us write for a living and all of us write for the love of it. So, it's important to say at the outset that writing is fantastic for your health. Here are some of the reasons why.

(1) Writing is therapy

I've written journals since I was an angst-ridden 15-year-old, desperate to figure out boys and God and school work. Pretty much in that order!

When I got divorced at 28, I worked out my rage and hurt on the page, writing reams of self-destructive words that slowly healed the pain inside. When I read those journals now, I don't even recognize myself, because I left that life behind as I wrote it out of my heart.

Writing can help you process grief or abuse, anger and pain. It can take the parts of your life that you need to deal with and become a counselor without you ever having to speak a word to another person. It can be your hidden therapist, and those words never need to be shared, or published, unless you want to turn them into a memoir at some point. Writing can heal you and help others if you share your journey.

"Writing can be cathartic and allows the writer to focus on something positive. It can almost be considered to be a mechanism for de-stressing and works well with mindfulness techniques."

AJ, The Healthy Writer survey

(2) Writing helps you process situations and learn about yourself

I write to figure out what I think about the world. In fact, I don't usually know what I think until I write about it, as the page gives me space to consider all the angles. I've written in my journals about whether I should move countries, about whether I should leave my job, and the doubts and fears that inevitably slam into life over the years. I've shared excerpts from my journals in this book and also in *The Successful Author Mindset*, where I bare my soul about the psychological reality of the writer's journey.

In my fiction, I write to delve deep into darker themes. My novel, *Desecration*, is a murder-mystery but also weaves in my thoughts on the meaning of the physical body, both in life and after death. In *Delirium*, I consider suicide and the spectrum of mental health we all move up and down in our lives. These are deep issues that can affect us all, and only through writing can I deal with them in a healthy way.

My friend and creative mentor, Orna Ross, teaches F-R-E-E writing: Fast, Raw, Exact and Easy. Write by hand as fast as you can without self-censoring. Lose control and don't think. Just write. It's incredible what comes out when you write like this and in the mess, there will be gold.

(3) Your writing can help other people, and that helps you

Writing is magic – or telepathy. It's two brains connecting over time and space, a way to reach another mind through the shapes of letters on a page. If you write about your own pain, you can help heal someone else's. You can change their mind, perhaps even change the course of their life.

All of us have books that changed our lives. In turn, your words can help other people, and it is (mostly) human nature to want to help others, so it will intrinsically reward you too.

(4) Writing can make you more optimistic

People who are more grateful have a positive, optimistic approach to life. They appreciate what they have, in terms of possessions and also, importantly, their social relationships. How do you become more grateful? Writing has an answer and the results are based in solid neuropsychological evidence.

University of California psychologists Emmon and McCullough ran an experiment in 2003. Participants wrote down five things for which they were grateful: the kindness of a friend, a beautiful view or just a sunset. They only had to write a sentence and they only had to do it once a week. The results were startling with clear improvements in well-being even for people with serious medical problems.

Using a gratitude journal can reduce your anxiety. It can help you move away from negative thoughts, especially when we live in a time of constant media negativity. There is an important connection between your thoughts and your emotions. Writing can make you more optimistic, and people who are more optimistic are happier.

(5) Writing can boost your physical health

The benefits of writing go beyond just improving your mood and making you more optimistic.

Emmon and McCullough also found that people who completed the gratitude tasks slept better. Losing sleep raises your blood pressure and makes you more susceptible to infections. Psychologists in Manchester in the UK have gone on to confirm that people who were more grateful slept longer and had better quality sleep. As psychologist Emmon put it: "if you want to sleep then count your blessings and not sheep."

There are other small studies that have suggested that expressive writing can have direct effects on physical health. This includes one study that suggested improved wound healing in people who were writing regularly. This could all be linked back to the positive effect of sleep, but there may be other factors at play. There are plausible bio-mechanisms for this, as long-term stress is known to trigger the release of hormones like cortisol. Having too many of those sloshing around will have effects that include damaging your body's ability to fight off infection.

(6) Writing helps you connect with others and build a community

Back in 2006, when I started writing seriously for publication, I didn't know any writers. I had no creative friends and I felt isolated and alone.

I started blogging in 2008 and by putting my words out into the world, I started to meet other writers. I went along to blogging meet-ups and connected with other writers on Twitter and then in real life. My writing was the catalyst that led me into an international community of creatives, and many of my best friends now are people I met online *because* of my blog. It continues to help others, but it also helps me connect.

(7) Writing helps you achieve your goals

I've always been a chronic goal-setter, and so I've always written down my goals in journals. I wrote an affirmation back in 2006, "I am creative, I am an author." This was before I'd even written or published anything. I couldn't even say it out loud. I kept it on a card in my wallet, whispering it in my mind while I walked to the train, commuting to the dreaded cubicle farm every day. After a few months, I began to say it out loud, then wrote it into my journal every night, while I took action in the daytime, writing what became my first book, *Career Change*.

That affirmation became reality a few years later, and I started my website, The Creative Penn, in December 2008. My next written goals were around income from the new business and then around leaving my day job, which I did in September 2011.

I continue to write down my goals every year, some I share on my blog and others I keep private in my journals. But I write them all down, because I know the process works, embedding the future reality in my mind as I take action toward it.

> While looking for a journal entry about headaches, I happened upon some ten year goals I had written in 2007: "In January 2017, I will be a full-time writer making a six-figure income."

The Joanna Penn who wrote that was still trapped in the day job. She had not even considered writing a novel. She had no website, no blog, no social media, no email list, no audience, not even one book out in the world. That was the year when the Kindle and the iPhone were launched, so the technology that powers much of my business now didn't even exist.

And yet, what I wrote down has come to pass.

"By recording your dreams and goals on paper, you set in motion the process of becoming the person you most want to be. Put your future in good hands — your own."

Mark Victor Hansen

Questions:

- Why do you write? Why is writing great for your physical and/or mental health?

Resources:

- Joanna's favorite journals: Moleskine or Leuchtturm A5 plain paper

- *The Five Minute Journal*, if you need guidance for gratitude. Recommended by Tim Ferriss and others.

- *The Artist's Way* - Julia Cameron. A classic book for creatives that includes the concept of Morning Pages, when you use journaling to empty your mind

- *F-R-E-E Writing* with Orna Ross, part of the *Go Creative* series of books and workbooks

Part One: The Unhealthy Writer

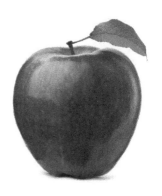

1.1 Stress, anxiety, burnout

You're feeling guilty because you haven't written anything this week.

You know that A.N. Other writer is making far more money than you and seems to be able to write so much faster – why can't you be that good?

You're behind on your writing goals or coming up against a publishing deadline and you have to get this thing written.

You're struggling for money so you need to get books out there.

Or you can't spare the time for your writing because you're working so hard.

You're snappy and angry and annoyed.

Your family don't understand why you're spending so much time writing when it doesn't make you happy and they put pressure on you to do less of it.

Your sleep is suffering because you're worried about all the things you should be doing.

You're trying to blog, write guest articles, do social media, master advertising and connect with other writers, as well as writing books. There's never enough time to do it all.

You're not making progress and you don't know what to do.

Do any of these thoughts sound familiar?

One of the reasons that we become writers is to live a different kind of life, a more creative life, more fulfilling and hopefully, a healthier life. But the incredible opportunities available to authors now have turned out to be a mixed blessing.

Writers are focusing on productivity and word count, on a book a month, feeding the hungry algorithms and the voracious appetite of readers. There's a constant stream of social media notifications that urge us to write more and faster, stoking the machine that provides cash flow as well as an ego boost.

Then there's the marketing side, all the things that you could be doing to get your books into the hands of readers, the technical stuff around categories and keywords and algorithms, and the sociable aspects like social media and blogging, as well as events and conventions. There are so many things that you *could* be doing right now. So, many authors are doing more and more and they're not taking a breath and they're getting stressed and burning out.

Part of the reason for me to write this book is to reflect on how I've fallen into some of these traps myself.

My husband, Jonathan, even said to me the other day, "You're the Creative Penn, not the Productive Penn. Take a break."

We all need to stop, take a step back and think about what we want for our lives in a holistic sense.

Burnout happens in the writer community when we forget why we're doing this in the first place. We bury the joy of creation in all the things that have to be done, or specific sales and ranking goals, or we write in a genre we don't really love, and some end up quitting writing all together.

"When I first started writing, it was therapeutic, like an escape from reality. But now it feels like a burden and I don't know how to get back the good feelings."

Alexa, The Healthy Writer survey

One of the reasons I left the corporate world was to change my life in a physical way, to be more healthy, hoping to add years onto my lifespan by removing bad stress and living a life I really wanted.

I burned out several times in that career, lurching from day to day powered by caffeine tablets, sugar and alcohol, until I had to leave the job in order to take a break. I didn't think the same existence would be possible for writers, but I've seen it in the community.

Because writing is hard work.

Sure, it's not physically hard but your brain uses a lot of energy and we have not evolved to spend hours a day trying to produce words from our heads. But there is a difference between being tired and feeling fatigued, stressed and on the way to burnout. Here are some distinctions.

Stress

"Reality is the leading cause of stress among
those in touch with it."

Lily Tomlin

Stress can happen in any job, even one that is supposedly an ideal occupation. The myth of the writer sitting in a gilded salon with Gauloise and black coffee in hand, writing perfect words while a publicist does all the heavy lifting is (sadly) indeed a myth.

Writing is intense work in a deeply satisfying way but it takes its toll as much as any job – especially if we lose the passion, the reason why we started writing in the first place, replacing that with deadlines and writing books we don't care about.

The idea of work-life balance springs from doing work that is not integrated with your life. Certainly, I used to think about balance when I worked as a business consultant, because my day job was not something I thought about out of hours or on weekends. It was something I did to pay for the rest of my life.

But being an author is all-encompassing and as a full-time writer, I don't separate my work from my life anymore.

The two are so entwined, and that is wonderful in one way as I am doing what I love. But it can also be the basis of burnout as there is no reason to ever stop working.

I'm an even-tempered, naturally happy and optimistic person. So if I find myself snappy, negative or persistently unhappy for days at a time, annoyed at the slightest thing, then I know something is wrong.

Stress is the feeling that everything is too much. You are juggling things and just about managing, but you're on the edge of collapse if you push too much further.

Of course, there are good types of stress. The edge of trying something new that pushes us outside our comfort zone. That might be a new writing technique, a different point of view, or going deep into a topic that might be uncomfortable.

On a physical level, when I did a double ultra-marathon, 100km in a weekend, the physical stress pushed me way past my comfort zone. I finished the course weeping with pain but the achievement of the goal was worth it. I feel the same way when working hard to finish a book sometimes.

Humans need stress in some way or we wouldn't achieve so much. We need to push ourselves beyond what we're comfortable with. But the problem comes when that stress goes on too long, when it stops us sleeping or when, over time, it leads to destructive behaviors like drinking or eating too much.

Back when I had a day job in the corporate world, there were constant project deadlines that were often impossible to reach, accompanied by stressful status meetings, even though it seemed that the deadlines were arbitrary and there was always another project right behind the one I focused on.

Financial stress is common, and family stress might be another issue. If you have young children at home, or you're a full-time carer, the level of stress is qualitatively different to the stress someone might feel in an office job with project deadlines, but it's no less real.

> "The greatest weapon against stress is our ability to choose one thought over another."
>
> *William James*

So how do you know when stress is getting too much?

When tiredness becomes fatigue

Being physically or mentally tired is completely normal at the end of a day when you have worked hard or done some physical activity. If you're not tired, what are you doing with your life?

But fatigue is waking up tired every day, with a deep exhaustion that seems to pervade your bones. It's like layer upon layer of tiredness, like a chronic syndrome, where every day you wake up feeling heavy and spend your whole day feeling more than tired.

It can be associated with other conditions, so definitely consult a medical professional if you're concerned, but it can also be down to persistent stress and overwork.

When I gave up my day job back in 2011 to become an author-entrepreneur, it took me a few months to get over the fatigue of constantly working in that toxic environment for so long. Some nights, I would sleep for 11 hours as I caught up on 13 years of sleep deprivation and overwork.

Anxiety

> "Anxiety is the handmaiden of creativity."
>
> *T.S.Eliot*

Anxiety can take many different forms. It can be a persistent low level of worry and concern that disturbs your sleep and may progress into mood issues like depression. Being unable to control that worry is often a marker of anxiety ramping up. You might feel restless and irritable.

Some people will get symptoms such as their heart racing and feeling sweaty or shaky, or it can kick off gut or digestive issues. Others may get panic attacks where they feel they can't breathe or that they are being choked and their throat is closing up.

If anxiety is severe, then see a medical professional, but low-level anxiety is common and we'll talk more about mood and mental health later in Chapter 1.15.

Burnout

There are three major components to burnout.

Emotional exhaustion (feelings of being exhausted and overextended by your work); depersonalization (a feeling of being removed and separate from various aspects of your life); and personal accomplishment (an absence of the feeling of accomplishment which may also be characterized by feelings of incompetence).

Creative work is often emotionally draining, and while it is normal to feel a certain level of exhaustion after the end of a project, you might be approaching burnout if these feelings are persistent and continue for months or even years after you've finished a book.

The domain of personal accomplishment will be particularly important to writers who suffer from self-doubt and Imposter Syndrome.

Imposter Syndrome is the feeling that whatever you do is never quite good enough, could always be better, and the persistent nagging sensation that your writing is terrible. Even when you have enjoyed some commercial and critical success, Imposter Syndrome will often remain as you wait for someone to pull back the curtain, Wizard of Oz style, and expose you as a fake and a phony.

This can result in symptoms such as irritability, anxiety, and difficulty concentrating. There may be other physical symptoms such as teeth grinding, palpitations, or headaches. There might be increased anxiety or trouble sleeping.

"If you feel burnout setting in, if you feel demoralized and exhausted, it is best, for the sake of everyone, to withdraw and restore yourself. The point is to have long-term perspective."

Dalai Lama

Managing stress, burnout, and anxiety

Part 2 goes into detail on many of these aspects, but these issues are so prevalent in the writer community that we wanted to make sure you had some action points upfront!

(1) Acknowledge your feelings and where you are right now

We like to think we're super-human, but everyone experiences these periods of stress and overwhelm, and many of us progress through levels of anxiety to burnout. The first step is to recognize the symptoms and acknowledge that you have a problem. Then you can look at ways to fix it, or at least manage it.

(2) Get organized

If you're feeling overwhelmed, it's a good idea to write down everything you think you should be doing so you can begin to organize it all.

I use two tools to manage the bulk of my life these days: Google Calendar and Things, a list-making app which syncs between my Mac and iPhone. Of course, there are many tools you can use, but if you have a calendar for scheduling and a To Do list app, you can manage pretty much everything. Of course, you can use paper for the analog option!

Start by writing down everything in your head until you can't think of anything else that needs doing. This can include personal and work tasks as well as writing tasks.

Once it is all out of your head, you can then start to organize and put specific dates when things are due. This will help you see what is urgent, what can wait and could be deleted. You can set recurring tasks and move dates if you get too busy. If I keep moving a task forward, I consider whether I should just delete it. Is everything on the list really so important?

I've also started scheduling downtime into my calendar. That might sound extreme, but without doing this, I end up constantly over-scheduling myself because I think I'm super-human! I've made the whole of December a downtime period with no speaking, podcast interviews, or external commitments, because I know my energy and mood are lower in the winter. I need to curl up and recharge, ready for January, which is when I perk up again. I also schedule a week every month where I don't have external commitments either and try to book in holidays as I used to do when I had a day job.

Running your own author business can take over your whole life, and I certainly work more hours than I ever did in the day job, so scheduling breaks is critical to sustainability for the long term.

(3) Assess, eliminate, and outsource tasks

What is your definition of success?

What do you want your life to look like? What suits your personality?

You can't do everything, so these questions can help you work out what you should cross off your To Do list entirely and can be the most powerful way to reduce stress.

For example, if you are an introvert who doesn't enjoy speaking at events, then don't do it. Concentrate on internet marketing for your books. If you enjoy watching YouTube videos, then consider using video as your primary marketing activity, but if you prefer writing short stories, then do that instead. Identifying your preferences will help you cull your To Do list.

For example, I tried doing Facebook Live Video, considered by many to be a powerful marketing tool, but I would dread it beforehand and didn't particularly enjoy it while doing it, so I have eliminated that from my marketing list.

You can also outsource tasks if you have the budget. I used to do all my podcast work myself, but now I have someone doing the video, a sound technician doing the audio, and my virtual assistant doing the show notes and transcript formatting. This means my own time has gone from five hours per show down to two hours per show, making it much more sustainable.

What can you eliminate or outsource?

(4) Say 'no' more

There's a period of time when you are starting out when you say 'yes' to every opportunity because you don't know anyone and you're building your brand. But if you're stressed and overwhelmed and you no longer have time for writing, then you need to say 'no' more.

I'm talking to myself here, because I still struggle with saying no. I'm a people-pleaser, but I've also said yes to things only to find myself regretting them, wishing I was doing something else. So when you're asked to do something, or you are asking yourself to do more, then stop for a moment. Give yourself space to consider it. Don't reply to that email immediately. Don't say yes before you've slept on it.

Do you really, really, really want to do this?

> "If you're not saying 'HELL YEAH!'
> about something, say 'no.'"
>
> *Derek Sivers*

(5) Try a digital fast

The internet is amazing.

It's the reason we can actually make a living as writers and reach readers all over the world. One study even found that people would rather have the internet than have sex, chocolate or alcohol. So it's an important part of our social and business lives as writers – but it can also be the cause of much stress.

If you check the news too much, you can be crippled by fear and anxiety about the state of the world. If you check Facebook or Twitter or Instagram all the time, you might feel comparisonitis at all the successful authors doing better than you, or feel like you're missing out on various conferences, holidays or promotions. And all of it makes us feel as if we can never do enough and we are always behind.

There is an answer to internet overwhelm. Turn it off!

Sounds simple but I know it's not easy. I am tethered to my iPhone just as much as many others.

But I do have periods of digital fasting, where I deliberately turn my phone to airplane mode. I take my phone on long weekend walks because it's also my fitness tracker, but I don't check email or social media. If I do longer trips, like cycling in India or walking in Europe, I only check it once a day. I took Facebook off my phone a month ago and feel a lot better without its daily tyranny.

We don't watch the news on TV, and I really recommend you wean yourself off that if you're struggling with stress. I monitor the headlines on the Financial Times or The Guardian news app, but the written word is less sensational than the TV announcements, which are designed to spike your interest and make you want to keep watching.

What you feed your brain has a huge impact on your mental health, so turn off the news and you'll feel a lot better!

(6) Breathe

Pay attention to your breath right now.

Where is it in your body? Can you direct it into your belly? Or your back? Or into the pain you're feeling?

Can you slow your breath to inhale for a count of five, hold it, and then exhale for a count of five?

These exercises may sound simple, but being aware of your breathing and taking time to just sit (or lie) and breathe is one of the most powerful, yet under-used, relaxation techniques. Because who has time to sit and breathe? There's always more to do.

When things used to get too much at work and I would be hyper-stressed, I would hold my breath, skip-breathing, yet unaware of it. Jonathan would put his arms around me and hold me against his chest and breathe with me, slowing our breath down together until I was calm again. I know parents who do this with their children and it really works, because you suddenly become aware of what your body is doing.

I tried meditation a number of times but always struggled to find the time – a classic case of the person who needs it the most and continues to resist it. The Headspace meditation app helped a little, but then I started to go to yoga several times a week to help my back pain, and breathing practice is part of those classes. It's now one of the main reasons I go. Time to breathe feels like a luxury, which is crazy, right?!

After a year of consistent yoga, I'm much more aware of my breath and realize that I tend to hold my breath or take shallow breaths when I'm stressed. Now I can feel when it is short and take steps to deepen and lengthen my breath in order to calm myself. It's helped me manage my stress, so if you're struggling, then consider incorporating breathing exercises into your daily routine.

(7) Develop a regular physical practice

Exercise helps to manage stress and anxiety. People who exercise regularly and are physical active have better health-related quality of life. There is also evidence that exercise can be used as a specific treatment to help manage anxiety.

A regular physical practice will help your body cope with long hours of writing and with emotional ups and downs. People who are physically fit are more resilient and able to cope with the stresses and strains of life. In Part 2, we'll look at some of the options that might help you in more detail.

(8) Consider a seasonal approach to your energy and creative patterns

Stress and burnout can happen because we try to achieve at the same level all the time, but that's just not natural.

Think about the rhythms of your energy, of your life. There are ups and downs, ebbs and flows with everything and that's the kind of cyclical and seasonal approach that can help us as creatives.

For example, during the period when I'm writing the first draft of a book, I will often work very hard. I will write almost every day for hours at a time, and I will get that first draft done. It's a very tiring period and I probably won't do much else other than write.

But then when that draft is finished, I stop and take a breather and start the editing process, which takes a different kind of brain power.

The preparation for a book can often take a lot of time thinking and plotting: not so much brute force creation of words, but the time it takes for the thinking and composting of ideas to occur. Later, there is launching and marketing, a different kind of energy again. Plus there are life events that happen, seasonal changes, so you can't expect to operate at the same level 100% of the time.

You need to allow for seasonal shifts, in your life, your location, and your creative projects.

There are big events that will occur that might be 'up' periods (e.g. birth of a child, wedding, moving house) and also problem times (divorce, death of a loved one, moving house, loss of a job).

Then there are the seasonal shifts in a year.

For the last few Decembers, I ended up talking to a friend about how terrible I was feeling and how down I was. Last year she said, "You realize that you're like this every December?"

Of course, I hadn't realized and I was being hard on myself, trying to maintain the same level of productivity in what is a down energy time for me. I don't like the end of the year, and England gets pretty dark over the winter.

But I love January. I love new beginnings. I love achieving things in the New Year.

So now I am being gentle with myself and allowing December to be fallow, a time of rest and reflection, and it's blocked out in my diary with *"Don't book anything"* for the whole month!

This type of cycle can also happen within the working week and within the day. There are times of the day when you're more energetic, more creative. Then there will be times when you dip.

You have to **learn your cycle and create within that cycle** rather than trying to brute force your way through, unless, of course, you're on a writing deadline.

But if we're thinking about burnout versus being sustainable in your creative life, then we have to be looking at practices and self-understanding, self-awareness that promotes a more healthy, creative life.

Questions:

- What is stressing you right now?

- Do you recognize any physical or mental symptoms of anxiety or even burnout? Write them all down even if they are not specifically related to your author life, as it is often the cumulative effect of everything that results in stress.

- What action can you take right now to reduce some of your stress or anxiety?

- Are you allowing for the seasonal shifts of day, week, time of year, time of life in your schedule? How can you factor that in more effectively?

Resources:

- The Worried Writer podcast with Sarah Painter
- Headspace app for meditation, mindfulness and breathing

1.2 Back, neck and shoulder pain

> "The typical seated office worker has more musculoskeletal injuries than any other industry sector worker, including construction, metal industry, and transportation workers."
>
> *Eric Jensen, quoted in* Deskbound: Standing Up to a Sitting World

Back pain. Everyone has it at some point.

I (Euan) have had recurrent problems with lower backache for years and years. Most of the time it doesn't give me any significant problems, but occasionally my lower back goes into spasm and I've suddenly found that my feet are unreachable. I can only gaze at them from a distance and touching them is an unimaginable reality. They may as well be on the Moon.

I've needed the help of my 10-year-old daughter to put on my socks, getting in and out of a chair is a major exercise, and driving has suddenly become a desperate challenge. I get a few days of my muscles squeezing in all the wrong places and then it relents. The muscles relax and it all goes back to normal.

I know I am in a permanent battle against my poor posture. I sit at work and I can feel myself curling over the desk. As I type this I'm forcing my shoulders back, trying to engage my tummy muscles. In another five minutes I'll be slumped over again, wondering why my lower back feels so stiff.

When it all gets too much and I feel like I'm 120 years old, groaning every time I stand up from my chair, I'll do a few exercises and stretches. I know there are ways to get my back feeling better, to unravel the knots, and regain mobility. It is hard to make it a habit but it is possible.

"Sitting in one position for hours, I guess it's inevitable, and even though I try to move around to prevent stiffness, it's easier said than done. That's the nature of writing, you get lost for hours and forget to move."

Becky, The Healthy Writer survey

Sitting, sedentary occupations and back pain

The evolutionary development of becoming a biped comes with some serious disadvantages in terms of our lower back. Unfortunately, in modern times, we've compounded the problem by becoming less active and then spending a huge amount of our time sitting down.

One of the reasons a sedentary lifestyle results in problems like lower back pain is due to physical deconditioning. Which is a polite way of pointing out that you are turning into a weak-limbed blob. The evidence is reasonably convincing that this happens in people with low back pain, though we do, as is often the case, have the old chicken and egg dilemma of causality. Did the deconditioning cause the back pain or did the deconditioning happen because of enforced inactivity due to back problems?

Whichever way this falls it doesn't matter too much in terms of management, because it's clear that **exercise helps low back pain**.

One thing is strongly shown in the evidence: if you have had low back pain in the past, you are nearly ten times more likely to get a recurrence in the following year. Other studies have shown similarly high recurrence rates.

So, if you are the kind of person who is getting pain, then prioritizing your back *now* is a worthwhile investment.

Mechanical low back pain

If you are getting low back pain or aches then chances are you have something known as mechanical low back pain. It's a catch-all term rather than one specific problem.

The back is a complex beast.

The bones are balanced on each other with multiple ligaments and muscles holding it all in the right place. When it starts getting a bit out of whack, then some muscles contract and you can quickly end up with pressure and spasm causing you pain.

Doctors talk about red flag signs and these highlight people who have something a lot more nasty than mechanical low back pain. Joanna mentions this in her description of the severe back pain she has suffered in the next chapter. Red flags include symptoms such as night-time pain, severe nerve pain, and any loss of control of the bladder or bowel.

The red flags are to try and pick up the tiny percentage of people with something more sinister than mechanical low back pain. It might be a slipped disc when the squishy cartilage between the vertebral bones protrudes and presses on the nerves as they leave the spinal cord. It might be another more serious problem where the bones themselves are diseased, perhaps through cancer or TB. If you have a red flag symptom, you definitely need to consult a healthcare professional.

Neck pain

Balancing our heavy heads with their giant homo sapiens brains on the top of our spines is a challenge. If you've ever suffered any kind of neck pain, the need for constant micro-adjustments to keep your head steady becomes painfully apparent. Rates of neck pain in office workers range from 42% to 69% in any given year.

That makes it incredibly common.

The evidence shows that people who are overweight are more likely to have problems with neck pain. Other studies have suggested that neck pain can be associated with slightly different factors, even such things as workplace bullying and sleep problems.

This might seem unrelated, but to a doctor this is a common way for some neck pain to present. It is a manifestation of stress. I certainly notice on my most stressful days that I hold myself with a ferocious tension and my shoulders slowly come up toward my ears. It is important to be aware of the cause as the management of that type of neck pain needs to be addressed differently.

"I recommend that people who spend long periods of time at their computer adopt a regular practice such as chi kung, tai chi, yoga, or whatever best suits them. Always check that your shoulders are relaxed and that you're neither slumping forward or back. Do shoulder/neck rolls to relax those areas."

CM Barrett, The Healthy Writer survey

Prevention of low back pain

One of the first things to do, if you can, is to avoid getting back pain in the first place.

We all know the truism that an ounce of prevention is worth a pound of treatment. Given the numbers of people suffering from low back pain, then you will be doing extraordinarily well if you avoid it, but it is absolutely a condition that comes and goes; it waxes and wanes in the vast majority of people.

The trick is that when you're enjoying a period when your back isn't bothering you, do something about it.

So, what can you do?

There has been a systematic review and meta-analysis into the prevention of low back pain. This is a scientific method to combine all the available research and it looked at a range of different options including strategies such as exercise, education, combining exercise and education, back belts, and shoe insoles.

They found that the best combination is **exercise in combination with education to reduce the risk of low back pain.**

Exercise on its own will reduce the risk as well. The evidence suggested that on their own, education, back belts, shoe insoles, and other ergonomic efforts probably don't do a huge amount to reduce episodes of low back pain.

The main challenges with any of these studies is the overall lack of high-quality evidence. That's a recurrent theme in almost all the studies that look into low back pain. The actual numbers suggest that exercise on its own could reduce the risk of a low back pain episode by about 35%. With exercise and education together that rises to a 45% reduction in risk of a low back pain episode. This was effective for up to a year but the effects reduce when past the one-year point.

You have to keep exercising to keep the risk of low back pain down.

That doesn't seem like a surprising finding, as it is not a one and done type of problem. You need to make long-term changes to your exercise habits to reduce the risk of back pain in the years to come.

Dynamic sitting, or wobbling around on a Swiss ball

There has been lots of research into how different seating options can help people with low back pain. There is a little bit of evidence that the use of a backrest can help in some circumstances, as can adjustable seat height and chairs which increase lordosis (those that make your lower spine arch backward more), so getting a good chair is a worthwhile investment.

There has been a lot of interest in the role of *dynamic sitting* or *active sitting*, using chairs, stools, or stability balls, where there has to be a constant amount of micro-adjustment in order for people to sit comfortably. If you've clocked someone wobbling away on a giant Swiss ball in front of their desk then you've seen them in action.

Gimmick or good evidence-based option?

A systematic review into these dynamic sitting methods found seven studies. The results were variable and the single randomized controlled trial that had a decent length of follow-up didn't find any significant reduction in low back pain. So, not much to go on there. I'd say they are worth a try if you are game. Joanna talks about how she uses a Swiss ball in the next chapter, and in Part 2 we'll cover ergonomics and improving your workspace as well as more help for your back.

"Being seated for so many hours a day has led to on and off shoulder, arm, and leg pain, which I've solved to a great extent with a desk that can go from standing to seated to standing again several times during the day."

Shelley Sperry, The Healthy Writer survey

Questions:

- Do you suffer from back, neck or shoulder pain?

- How much is this pain interfering with the quality of your life? How would you feel if it carried on like this for the rest of your life?

- When does this get particularly bad? Can you identify physical postures that make it worse or better?

Resources:

- See Chapter 2.1 for more on improving your work space and Chapter 2.5 on how to sort out your back.

- *The Back Sufferer's Bible* by Sarah Key. Also resources at www.simplebackpain.com

1.3 A personal journey to a pain-free back

Ask any writer what hurts, and many will say it's all about back, neck and shoulder pain.

I worked in the corporate world for 13 years as a cubicle slave, and back pain and headaches were always a problem. After all, we're not meant to sit down all day, hunched over a desk, typing or writing. It's just not what we are meant to do as humans.

When I left my job to become a full-time author-entre-preneur, my hours in the chair expanded. I was writing more, but there was also email, social media, and all the associated admin work that goes along with being a writer.

About a year into writing full-time, the pain got so bad that I was waking at night, unable to sleep because my lower back was keeping me awake. I was popping painkillers every day just to keep functioning. When I (finally) went to the doctor, he said that the night pain was a red flag and immediately sent me for tests, especially as there are spinal tumors in my family history.

It was a worrying time, but I had the scans, and everything was fine. There wasn't anything wrong with me, so they sent me to the physiotherapy team, who gave me some exercises to do. They weren't very effective, but at least it began my journey to a pain-free back, and five years later, I am almost pain-free – if I keep up the maintenance.

Here are the things I've done to get rid of the pain and live a more functional life.

Ergonomic assessment at my home office

Those of you who have worked in the corporate world will know of the ergonomic assessment. Someone comes around to your desk and moves your chair up and down and takes pictures and gives suggestions. To be honest, I'd never taken it that seriously when I worked in my previous company, but this time I was very motivated, and you can hire someone who can come around to your house to set up your home office as a freelancer.

At the time, I was just using a basic office chair and a laptop on a desk with a couple of books underneath and a wireless keyboard. Of course, I work in cafés as well, but if you know the principles, you can apply them wherever you are. These are the changes I made out of that first assessment which might also help you.

Screen height

If you're using a laptop, get a stand for it so your eyes are level with the top of the screen. Check the position of your neck, as if you are looking down too much, your neck muscles are hyper-extended and there's pressure on your shoulders and arms. Use a separate keyboard so you can have your arms at the right level.

Sit / stand desk

I moved from a static desk to a desk that moves up and down. Two years later, the motor broke down so I now use a wooden 'topper' which I know will never break down!

(Mine is from StandStand.com.) There are also portable options so it can be used in cafés if you don't mind looking a bit weird. I do all my podcasting standing up, whether it's my own show or other interviews, so I probably do 1-2 hours most weekdays standing up.

Swiss ball

This won't be for everyone, but I moved from a chair to a Swiss ball, which has several benefits. It's wobbly so you have to make micro movements to stay on the ball which keeps the back mobile. You can also lean back and stretch while thinking about things or taking micro-breaks. I've found that the most important stretches for me are reversing the hunch by leaning back over the ball and raising my arms over my head, so I do that several times a day.

Go ambi-mouse-trous

I'm not sure that's a real word, but being ambidextrous with a mouse can be useful if you are getting pain in your wrist, elbow or arm in general, as it could be the beginnings of repetitive strain injury (RSI) or even carpal tunnel. I got a left-hand mouse and learned to use it so I could shift between one hand and the other to lessen the pain in my right forearm.

I was also going to the gym and taking walking breaks, which all helped a little, but after two years, I was still getting pain.

We often put up with pain because we think it's normal, an acceptable part of the job. But it's not acceptable. We don't have to just live with the pain. There are things we can do to make our writing lives easier and more sustainable.

Physiotherapy

I went to see a new physio. After examining me, she said that the RSI in my arm was not so much my mouse or anything like that. It was tension in my back, so we started to work on functional movements. If you've been to a physio, you'll know it can be a painful process, but it loosened things up, and I had periods without pain. I learned stretches that would help me keep the pain in check, and I started walking more regularly and for longer. But the pain still hadn't gone away completely, and I didn't want to rely on regular physio, so I looked for other options.

Walking

I've always enjoyed walking and started to increase the length of my walks as I focused on my physical health. When we moved to Bath, I added in a longer walk every Sunday, as when I'm at home, I tend to work all the time – the dangers of a home office! So getting out the house helped in multiple ways. Now I do a regular 4-5 hour walk every week, as well as longer multi-day walking holidays and ultra-marathons, detailed further in Chapter 2.12. The physical exertion of walking longer distances refreshes me in so many ways and is now an important part of my life.

Walking is great, but it's not stretching and can actually add pain in the back, so I needed something more.

Yoga

I had tried yoga a number of times before, usually at the gym, but I'd always felt out of place. I'm not a slender Instagram-yoga-body woman, so I felt clumsy and had given it up every time I'd tried over a period of around eight years. It had never stuck, but so many people recommended yoga as a sustainable practice for back pain that I was ready to try again.

This time I went to a yoga school, an actual place dedicated to different forms of yoga, not a gym where it was one of many classes on offer. I started with gentle yoga, aka the remedial class, which was full of people like me, of all different ages, who could barely move. At that point, I couldn't sit cross-legged, even on a number of blocks and I found it difficult to bend over and touch my feet, one of the basic aspects of the sun salutation. There were a *lot* of functional problems with my body.

But as I started to go to these gentle yoga classes, the pain began to lessen significantly, and my RSI disappeared. As I progressed to the normal classes and increased the number of times I went, my pain almost completely disappeared.

Yoga has been a miracle for me and is now an integral part of my life, for the physical movement aspect and maintenance of my body, but also for the space to breathe. If you want to try it, then I recommend you go to a specific yoga school rather than a gym, because they will have sessions that will suit you as a beginner.

One of the marvels of yoga is the spinal twist, which, if you don't know any yoga, is not as painful as it sounds. There are various forms, and the simplest one can just be lying on your back with your knees going in one direction, and your upper body and head turned in the other direction. I crave this posture now and do it at home as well as in class. If I don't do yoga for more than a week, I feel the pain coming back, so it is part of my life now, a practice just as much as writing.

So that's my journey to an almost pain-free back.

It's been incremental and requires ongoing maintenance, but by focusing on solving the problem, I now have a huge improvement in functional movement and my mental health has improved with yoga and walking. I also rarely take painkillers these days.

Don't settle for the pain.

Your journey to becoming pain-free will be different to mine, but you *can* take steps to improve it. It may take years of experimentation, but it's worth it, and you might find a new hobby/lifestyle along the way!

1.4 Repetitive Strain Injury (RSI)

Writers are at high risk of RSI, and for any author the consequences of developing pain while writing are worrying. If that pain stops you from using your computer, then it becomes very serious.

Certain groups of people are more prone to RSI. Anyone doing a repetitive task can be at risk. Sometimes it is factory workers who are doing repetitive jobs on production lines, or it can be musicians, or someone working on a checkout in a supermarket. It could appear from too much DIY or activities like golf. Heavy computer users are definitely on the list.

It is possible to get RSI in all sorts of areas but writers are usually troubled in the hands and wrists. Sometimes you can run into problems with relatively short periods of typing and this often reflects poor posture and awkward positioning. It could also be due to intense bursts of activity without adequate rest.

Pain is a common symptom but this can come in various hues. It might be more of a throbbing or aching pain and there could be stiffness, weakness or cramp. It is possible you might get swelling and soreness in the affected areas and the pain can start to cause problems even when you are not doing the activity.

RSI can be split down into two main varieties, the imaginatively named type 1 and type 2.

Type 1 RSI

Type 1 RSI has an obvious and specific diagnosis. Carpal tunnel syndrome is the classic example.

Type 1 problems will often involve some kind of inflammation and irritation of the tendons. Tendons are what the muscles turn into before they attach to various bits of bone but they also have a covering, a tendon sheath, that can get inflamed as well. Inside that sheath is some slippery joint liquid known as synovial fluid. It is there to reduce the friction and keep us moving without squeaking. Irritation in here is known as tenosynovitis. By and large, humans don't appreciate friction when they move and no one likes to feel friction when they are simply wiggling their fingers over a keyboard.

Carpal tunnel syndrome

This is a problem where the nerve that passes through your wrist doesn't quite have enough space. It gets squeezed and you then get pain and numbness over certain fingers – usually the thumb, index finger, middle finger and sometimes half the ring finger. The pain can be severe and it can travel back up the arm as well. And, if you get it on one side then there is a much greater risk that you will get it on the other side as well.

Carpal tunnel syndrome is relatively easy to diagnose from the symptoms described. Clinical examination will help confirm it and often there is no need for further investigations, although sometimes people do get sent for nerve conduction studies.

Treatments include measures such as wrist splints and trying to avoid activities that make it worse. If it persists, you might need to have an operation that can relieve the pressure. Either way, it might be worth heading straight over to the dictation section in Chapter 2.7. You'll get a lot of benefit if you can include dictation in your workflow.

"Many things can cause repetitive strain injuries but in my case the problem was hours of keyboarding and data entry at a workstation that did not properly or ergonomically support my body mechanics."

Marianne Sciucco, from an article on
RSI written for TheCreativePenn

Type 2 RSI

This is where it can get a whole lot more nebulous and varied. The symptoms with type 2 RSI will be very different from one person to the next. This makes it harder to diagnose as well.

You may get all of the various symptoms of aching, cramp and numbness, etc. There is some evidence that RSI can be associated with stress and this may simply be due to the muscular tension that often comes with it. So, if you get asked about stress, it doesn't mean your doctor thinks it is all in your head. Neck pain and some headaches can have a similar background, and tackling stress and tension is an important element of managing the problem.

Getting to the diagnosis can be a messy business as the more distinct type 1 RSIs are gradually excluded.

Strategies to manage RSI

You may get told to stop doing whatever triggers it. That can be scary if it is a suggestion to stop writing. It is, however, almost always the right answer to some degree.

In reality, if things haven't gone too far, you will not have to stop all typing or computer use, but *you are going to have do things a bit differently*. Keeping on the same path is not a good option. It is not the type of problem that will go away without some kind of change.

Some of the type 1 RSIs will have specific treatments such as steroid injections and, in some cases, surgical options. Those are unlikely to be on offer in type 2 RSI.

If you can catch the pain of RSI early then with adjustments it is possible to reduce the impact and steer a route around it. If you plow on with a 'no pain-no gain' mentality then it is possible to set up a very nasty chronic condition that will martyr you for years.

Ergonomics and RSI

The whole topic of ergonomics is huge, but a holistic approach to RSI can pay dividends. See Chapter 2.1 for more ways to improve your work space.

It is highly probable that if you are having issues with RSI you will have linked problems in your neck, back, and even your legs. You might be something of a bio-mechanical crock. If you spend large chunks of your life hunched in a certain position then the knock-on effects should not be underestimated.

Laptops and RSI

There is good evidence that notebooks are particularly bad news when it comes to RSI. They are the ergonomic equivalent of smoking 20 cigarettes a day. Well, OK, they won't kill you but they can certainly make you feel like killing someone else.

We contort our hands and wrists into all sorts of twisted postures to use them effectively. The screen is at the wrong height and your wrists are cocked at a weird angle. The ambience of a coffee shop may do wonders for your productivity, but using your laptop is likely to be smashing you from the ergonomic perspective. One study with university students found benefit in using an adjustable chair or notebook riser when these were used in combination with some ergonomic training.

If you are using a notebook at home then consider getting yourself an external keyboard. You may resent the additional cost but it is a worthwhile investment in your long-term health. Put your notebook on a riser. This raises the notebook up to a more comfortable angle for screen viewing.

Physiotherapy and physical treatments

Do some exercises. These could be simple core strengthening exercises or gentle stretches. Joanna has described how yoga has made a huge difference to her RSI and back pain in Chapters 1.3 and 2.6.

It is likely that yoga is having its effects through several different mechanisms. It can build general fitness, and it will improve flexibility as well as muscular strength. Your core muscles will get stronger. And, the mindful elements of yoga may help you relax and reduce tension. Even the breathing techniques can be usefully used during the working day to help your mindset. There is a lot going for yoga!

Dictation

For obvious reasons, dictation will immediately help people with RSI. It's perfectly clear that dictating will give your hands a rest as you don't have to use them at all. Even better, with the use of portable recording devices including smartphones and dictaphones, it is possible to add to your step count while doing it. You can get some fresh air if you want, and Joanna takes walks down by the canal. Heck, you can just use a long lead on your microphone and pace around your office.

Dictation is particularly effective for the production of first drafts. It won't work so well for editing. See Chapter 2.7 for more details on how you can get going with dictation.

Questions:

- Are you getting pain from any period of writing or typing?

- Is your posture and your work space putting you at risk of RSI?

- What can you do to reduce the risk of RSI? Are you using an external keyboard and riser with a laptop?

- Do you take regular breaks from your writing? Are you doing any physical exercise that will build your resilience and reduce the chance of RSI?

Resources:

- The chapters on workspace, sorting out your back, dictation, exercise and more in Part 2 will give you more ideas. You should also be able to find RSI assessment professionals near you.

1.5 Writing with chronic pain

"Henry VIII was in chronic pain. I know what that does to degrade the personality, to detract from rationality, and I think I can write about this well."

Hilary Mantel talking about Bring up the Bodies

Hilary Mantel, twice Booker Prize winner, has spoken about her struggles with chronic pain from endometriosis and the role writing has played in helping her. She had a long process where diagnosis of her condition was delayed.

If you look at the evidence, the success rates for treatment of people with chronic pain are disappointingly low. There are no easy answers, but the best management seems to lie with a genuinely holistic approach that treats each patient individually and works with them across a range of options. There is an increasing recognition within medicine that chronic pain (whatever the cause) should be treated as a disease state in its own right and that there are multiple factors in play.

It can't simply be fixed with a prescription. There are clear dangers with past policies where there has been far too much emphasis on prescribing and the use of opioid medications. However, many people do get relief from medications as well and they are undoubtedly part of a comprehensive approach.

"There really is a trick to the writing while chronically ill. But the trick is personal, and it's tailored to each individual person … The word *management* is the key. The other key is *acceptance*. (I have a tougher time with the second one.)"

Kristine Kathryn Rusch, writing on her blog, KrisWrites.com, about her chronic migraines.

Medication and chronic pain

The consequence of low success rates with medication is that it has had a ratchet effect on prescribing. Every time a medication doesn't work then the doctor turns to the next medication up the scale. This has been reinforced by a model taught to students and doctors known as the World Health Organization 'pain ladder' that works well for acute pain. This sensibly encourages us to start with medications with the fewest side effects. It also passes on a subliminal message that the answer to pain is to always keep going up through the gears. If a medication doesn't work, then simply try something slightly stronger.

The stronger medications all tend to be opioids. There is not great evidence for the effectiveness of opioids to control chronic pain – but some people do clearly benefit as well. In some cases it can worsen the situation due to a phenomenon known as opioid hyperalgesia where the opioids make the experience of pain *worse*. This means sometimes pain specialists will be able to help improve chronic pain by *reducing* opioid medication. This is tough and difficult territory. Individuals need careful assessment by experienced specialists and blanket proclamations on the best management can't be made.

What is known is that, of course, opioids have side effects, the most serious side effect being overdose that can result in death. There were 15,000 deaths in the USA in 2015 that were blamed on prescription opioid medication. It is thought as many as 1 in 4 people who have been prescribed opioids (for non-cancer pain) in the USA will struggle with addiction. That is a lot, but it can be turned on its head as well, as it suggests that three-quarters of people, the majority, don't have addiction problems with their opioid pain relief medication.

"Of pain you could wish only one thing: that it should stop. Nothing in the world was so bad as physical pain. In the face of pain there are no heroes."

George Orwell, 1984

Back, neck and shoulder pain

This is one source of chronic pain that is likely to be amenable to treatment. Similarly, problems with RSI fall into this category. While the occasional tablet can help with pain, the best long-term management for these conditions is likely to be some kind of physical therapy and changes to lifestyle and working conditions. These are discussed in Part 2.

Fibromyalgia

This is a long-term condition that is not yet well understood. Pain is an overwhelming feature but fatigue can also be a significant problem. The diagnosis is still clinical, meaning there are no specific blood tests or investigations that give the diagnosis. Doctors will look for tender trigger points in particular parts of the body and some blood tests might be done to exclude other possible diseases. At the moment, research points toward the benefits of exercise programs that gradually increase in intensity. Cognitive behavioral therapy may help some people as well.

The Netflix documentary *Gaga: Five Foot Two* gives an insight into how musician Lady Gaga manages her chronic fibromyalgia pain alongside her creativity. In September 2017, she canceled her European tour because of "severe physical pain" and continues to struggle with managing pain and trying to achieve her goals of helping people through her songs.

Nerve pain

Damage to nerves can result in neuropathic pain which is a particularly unpleasant experience. This is likely to need careful discussion with a healthcare professional and there are more exotic medication and sophisticated medical techniques like nerve blocks that could be considered. The medications certainly have their share of side effects and challenges and like any prescribing, the benefits need to be weighed against the risks.

Chronic pain needs a holistic approach

If you have chronic pain, a holistic approach is going to be helpful. You should cast the net wide here when it comes to managing your pain. Some of these options may be available in your healthcare service and some of them you can put in place yourself. Areas that are important:

Pharmacotherapy:

Getting your medications right, if needed, is important and will need careful discussion with a healthcare professional.

Physical activity:

This will be hugely dependent on the type of pain and problems you have but can be of enormous benefit.

Social interaction:

Finding a community, valuing your relationships with family, friends, and colleagues has good evidence to show the benefit. There may be value in building connections with people who have chronic pain and who have the same underlying problems. There are many support groups out there with people who will have a keen understanding of your daily struggles.

Physical treatments:

These could range from the simple use of heat packs to more complex interventions like the use of TENS machines or regular sessions with a specialist physiotherapist.

Diet and other lifestyle changes:

These shouldn't be under-estimated and, depending on the condition, can make a huge difference. Giving up smoking or reducing alcohol can be tough for people even without the burden of chronic pain, but with the right support can give obvious benefits.

Psychological therapies:

There are many of these and reviews of the evidence suggest that psychological therapies can be effective in helping people with chronic pain. Treatments like cognitive behavioral therapy (CBT) can reduce the depression and anxiety associated with chronic pain. They can also reduce the disability and catastrophic thinking that goes with it. However, only a few people will have the pain itself reduced and it's often more about the ability to cope with and live with the pain.

The cycle of catastrophic thinking with chronic pain can be really damaging. You may think thoughts like "I'm never going to get better" and "my life is over." It is, as Hilary Mantel put it, a degradation of the personality. These thoughts lead to negative emotions that can then fuel lower mood and increased anxiety. And these drive the cycle of catastrophic thinking onward. CBT is good at breaking down that cycle.

Writing with chronic pain

There is no sense in which having chronic pain is 'worth it.' Those people that have chronic pain, or have endured it, have gone deep into their personal reservoirs of spirit to cope. You may be able to use that for your writing and it will inevitably form part of your creative process. There are proven benefits in writing for all people and it is possible that in people with chronic pain those are even greater.

Author Angela Clarke has the degenerative connective tissue disorder Ehlers-Danlos III (EDS III), which, among other things, means she suffers from chronic pain. Here's how she manages her life as a writer.

"It's all about pacing. Writing as a career is marvelous, because you can control your time.

Start thinking about your body as your tool, the thing you need to protect and nurture in order to continue working. And so, build in what you need to keep that tool at its best. Redesign your routine so that it allows for the impact of your meds, so that you don't boom and bust, so that it includes regular breaks. For example, I write for a couple of hours and then visit my physio, then I'll have a nap, and when I'm refreshed, do a bit more work. That way I achieve more than if I'd forced myself to stay at my desk for a solid eight hours.

The thing with any chronic condition is to **never let your batteries run completely down.** You must stop, in order to keep going. It's at odds with the Terminator mentality that our society embraces and seems to celebrate, but ultimately, the Terminator is always defeated.

If you can adopt the balance needed to keep going, you may very well outstrip your colleagues who are currently healthy but doomed to burnout. **A chronic condition is a super-power** in that regard: it gives us a head start on understanding the importance and value of time."

Author Rebecca Bradley also recommends pacing:

"I live with a genetic condition that causes chronic and debilitating pain. As a writer, I find **pacing allows me to create and manage the pain I live with**. You will be surprised how much you can achieve by working for short periods of time and then taking a rest before returning to your task."

Questions:

- How does pain affect you?

- Could you explore more options to help manage your pain? Have you gone beyond medication and approached it from multiple angles?

- Are you getting into cycles of negative thinking around your pain and illness? Would you benefit from psychological help to break those down?

- How does chronic pain affect your writing?

Resources:

- See your local medical professional for issues related to chronic pain. There may also be in-person support groups locally or online for your particular situation.

1.6 Sedentary life and inactivity

"Sitting is more dangerous than smoking, kills more people than HIV and is more treacherous than parachuting … We are sitting ourselves to death."

Dr. James Levine, quoted in Deskbound: Standing Up to a Sitting World

Sitting is the new smoking.

As a doctor, working in primary care and family medicine, I see the consequences of inactivity all the time. The list of problems that could be eased from being more active is long: tension headaches, depression, asthma and other lung problems, any stress-related condition. Those are just a few.

And, for all the medicines in the world, changing your lifestyle is the most effective way to manage a huge proportion of the problems dealt with by family doctors.

A worldwide study published in the *Lancet* in September 2017 showed reductions in death and events like heart attacks and strokes at even modest levels of exercise. It didn't matter what you did or where you live, those findings held up across all countries. Higher levels of physical activity were even better.

For many people, the idea of getting more active remains a slightly nebulous wish, a vague goal that seems out of reach. It is tremendously difficult to change your lifestyle. Making the changes is not easy. And getting them to stick for the months and years needed to make a genuine impact is a challenge.

People are getting more overweight and that is bringing huge problems. Some of the dietary causes are still being hotly debated, but everyone would agree that we have an epidemic of inactivity. People simply don't come close to doing enough physical activity.

One thing that the phrase 'sitting is the new smoking' does is give people a nudge about their behavior. Perhaps it might give you pause for thought and consider whether your lifestyle is good for your health. Actually most people need a bit more than a nudge: a sharp elbow in their ribs is often helpful. Figuratively speaking.

If you haven't already worked it out then let me offer that sharp elbow. Get active.

Do more, move more. Find a way to integrate it into your life as a writer. If you are active, you will probably live longer. Forget about that, though, and concentrate on the immediate benefits.

There is no single better way to improve your quality of life right now.

"I'm on my butt more hours a day than I sleep."

Lynn Cahoon, The Healthy Writer survey

Specific research on sitting and physical activity

Some of the research around this can get a little confusing. This is immediately obvious when you consider a couple of jobs at the extremes of the spectrum. A coal-miner, who isn't going to spend any time sitting down, and is highly physically active, is likely to have considerably worse health outcomes than almost anybody else. Senior executive roles where people spend their entire lives sitting down live the longest.

We need to bear in mind that health is intrinsically bound up in all sorts of other factors that include whether you work for a living, where you live, what you eat, whether you smoke, and your social and family circumstances. People like CEOs may spend a lot of time sitting but they are also likely to be non-smokers, drink moderately, and exercise regularly. All of that counteracts the sitting.

A recent academic paper looked at all the research and whittled the studies down to eight systematic reviews covering 17 studies. They wanted to establish if sitting down and being inactive *caused* deaths. The definition of 'sitting' included general sedentary behaviors such as time spent watching TV and looking at screens. The review showed that there was a consistent pattern. Sitting was related in time to the causes of death.

The conclusion was clear: **sitting is killing people.**

Physical activity in the modern world

We do have a bonkers relationship with activity.

We spend our lives sitting in heated boxes, barely moving a few steps from one corner of the box to another. We eat and we hardly move. Then, we will occasionally leave our boxes and get into other metal boxes that drive us around. Sometimes, we get out of those boxes and go into another heated box where we run madly on the spot or jump up and down vigorously until we are sweaty. We then get back in our boxes, first the metal ones and then back to the brick ones. We then repeat this pattern.

We need to re-think how we engage with physical activity in this kind of modern environment.

Being inactive, spending too much time sitting down, and being sedentary in general will shorten your life. It will also erode the quality of your life. This is not some abstract notion where you might increase your life expectancy by an average of a few months at best. This is quite specifically related to health problems that you will have during the course of your normal life. Symptoms you can sit and list right now.

Being more active and taking breaks from sitting was the single most common tip in the Healthy Writer survey. For many writers there is a good chance that the problems you have can be improved by being more active.

Questions:

- How many hours are you sitting every day? How has that changed in the past few months or years?

- Can you list symptoms and problems that could be related to sitting?

- Has an increase in your time spent writing made you less active?

- What have you done to counteract the sedentary nature of writing?

Resources:

- Read Chapter 2.8 to start on the path towards being an active writer.

- *Deskbound: Standing Up to a Sitting World* – Kelly Starrett and Juliet Starrett

1.7 Sleep problems and insomnia

"Routinely sleeping less than six or seven hours a night demolishes your immune system, more than doubling your risk of cancer."

Matthew Walker, Why We Sleep:
The New Science of Sleep and Dreams

How do you feel about your sleep?

The distress that goes with losing sleep, having disrupted sleep, or just feeling that in some way your sleep is unsatisfactory results in a great deal of angst. People are increasingly preoccupied with sleep. Fair enough. Getting the right amount of sleep on a regular basis could be the single best life hack there is.

I'm a bit obsessive about sleep, too. I've a regular routine and my sleep suffers when I step out of that routine. Other than the occasional bout of jet lag, I've never suffered from insomnia but I've had my share of sleep deprivation so I'm no stranger to that discomfort. I've worked as a junior doctor, done countless on-call shifts where I've been dragged out of my bed in the middle of the night, and been part of rosters involving long stretches of nights and antisocial shifts. When I worked in the Emergency Department we used to work a series of shifts that included the dreaded 8pm- 4am.

I have children who came in a tight grouping and at one stage I had three children under three. There were years where I didn't get an unbroken night's sleep. I've been in the British Army, where sleep deprivation is regarded as a necessary element of any exercise to test out training. There's a reason for that: it's the single easiest way to ramp up the intensity of training and test your ability to function under duress.

I hate not sleeping. I find it easy to believe that shift work shortens your life. It is unspeakably stressful.

Some sleep basics

We go through different cycles while we sleep. Each of the cycles will last for something like 90-120 minutes. Typically the two main types are rapid eye movement sleep (REM) and non-rapid eye movement sleep (NREM). There are distinct physiological differences in things like your brain waves, eye movements, and muscle tone during each of these phases. Changes in NREM can be sub-divided into three different stages that are progressively deeper. In a typical night of sleep deeper NREM sleep tends to dominate at the start of the night and REM sleep is more common in the second half. As we age, we spend less time in the deeper stages of sleep and it is normal to wake up more often.

Sleep and resilience

Loss of sleep results in problems with using your brain, known as cognitive impairment. That's well-established. It has also been shown that we are not, ourselves, very good judges of that impairment. This is a worrying combination. There can be a strange kind of bravado associated with missing out on sleep, and the inability to realize that it damages how our brains function puts an interesting spin on this.

Evidence related to health and sleep deprivation

"Insomnia became the norm. I would lie down to try to sleep at a normal hour, but then it was like I had a tape in my brain that was on permanent fast forward and refused to shut off."

Halona Black, The Healthy Writer survey

What does it mean to not get enough sleep? What does it do to your body?

It slows up your cognition.

Putting it bluntly, it makes you a little bit more stupid than you otherwise would be.

It also dulls your reactions in the same way as drinking some alcohol. Even one night of disrupted sleep makes you more likely to have an accident driving the next day. Several nights without sleep will leave you feeling grotty. Sleep deprivation has a grisly history in its use as a form of torture.

There is a lot of evidence about the health effects of sleep. A reduction in the number of hours of sleep can have an impact on cardiovascular health, your risk of cancer, and your mental health. Obviously, this is fairly complex research and there are lots of conflicting and compounding factors. People who are ill often have worse sleep, and teasing them out of the research is difficult. The challenge with sleep is always working out whether it is causal or whether it is a symptom of some other problem.

There is evidence that prolonged periods of poor sleep or loss of sleep will result in increases in blood pressure. The wider health implications of prolonged periods of sleep loss or disruption are severe. Night shift work increases the risk of breast cancer and shift work of all kinds is associated with an increased risk of events such as heart attacks and strokes.

Tracking your sleep

As with so many things, monitoring and keeping a record is an important step toward working out what to do.

It can take any form you want, but the American Academy of Sleep Medicine has an example of a sleep diary format. A popular option these days is to use some kind of wearable technology such as a fitness tracker. These will usually tell you how long you have been asleep and will also provide little graphs of your sleep cycles including deep sleep, light sleep, REM sleep, and awake periods. We'll go into more ways to help your sleep in Part 2.

Questions:

- How much sleep are you getting every night? Do you feel that is enough for you? Are you going through life with a constant sleep deficit?

- How often do you wake up naturally without an alarm or interruption?

- Have you tracked or monitored your sleep?

Resources:

- American Academy of Sleep Medicine – 2 week sleep diary www.yoursleep.aasmnet.org/pdf/sleepdiary.pdf

- Sleep Junkies website – www.sleepjunkies.com

- *Why We Sleep: The New Science of Sleep and Dreams* – Matthew Walker

1.8 Eye strain, headaches and migraine

"I typically keep lubricating eye drops near my computer. I also get away from my computer screen for a bit when my eyes start hurting. Placing a cool wet washcloth over my closed eyes also helps."

Christa Geraghty, The Healthy Writer survey

Eye strain can be a significant problem for writers who stare at a computer screen for hours at a time.

We've all been there.

The gritty feeling that someone has sprinkled your eyes with sand. The effort to keep focused with the constant irritation of eyes that don't want to play anymore. If you wear glasses or have any visual impairment then you will hit problems at an earlier stage.

The impact of staring at screens has been explored by researchers for many years. It was first described back in 1973, and in the 1980s evidence emerged on the effects of prolonged exposure. If there is one thing that the research hasn't kept pace with, it is the astonishing increase in exposure to screens most people now have.

In one 1994 study the high-risk group were exposed to 'visual display terminals' (VDTs) for more than 20 hours *per week*. Tot up all the time you spend in front of a computer writing, add in the hours spent squinting at your phone, and then throw in some hours of television as well. Twenty hours of screen-time in a week would be regarded as low by many nowadays.

Even in the early 1990s, the explosion in screen-time for the average person could not have been predicted. It's crazy to think that the first iPad was only launched in 2010, but since then screens have become ubiquitous. The participants in the 'high risk' group in the 1994 study were around three times as likely to get problems with some kind of eye discomfort.

These included a whole range of symptoms that will be familiar to us: smarting, a gritty feeling, redness, and sensitivity to light. They also found that sitting closer to the screen was more likely to result in problems and people who wore glasses had greater difficulties.

How common are eye symptoms?

Modern studies have suggested that up to half of people using screens can get problems with their eyes.

One of the most recent studied 116 flat-screen users to explore the range of eye symptoms they experienced. In that sample, 23% suffered moderate to severe symptoms that included severely tired eyes, sensitivity to bright light, blurred vision, and general eyestrain or dry eyes. Symptoms were more common in females and worse in those who spent more than six hours per day looking at the screen.

Another study of 500 students in the United Arab Emirates found that over half suffered a burning sensation in the eyes and just under half suffered from tired eyes. They also found that females were more likely to be affected. When the screen was viewed from a distance of more than 50cm, headaches decreased by 38%.

"One issue that came up with my ophthalmologist is the fact that when people sit at their computers for an extended period of time, they tend not to blink as often. I now make sure to take a break every hour, to stretch, use saline drops and rehydrate."

Lydiae, The Healthy Writer survey

Why do screens cause problems?

One of the reasons people run into difficulty with the use of screens is around blinking.

One of the functions of blinking is to help lubricate our eyeballs. Blinking spreads tears over the surface in a thin but uniform layer. The tears help deliver oxygen as well as nutrients to our eyes. They also help protect against infection with an ingredient called lysozyme and heal any damage to the surface.

We normally blink at around 12 to 16 blinks per minute. That's one every five seconds. However, when we look at computer screens that reduces to a rate which can be as low as six blinks per minute. Just one every 10 seconds. We sit there wide-eyed as our eyeballs shrivel up.

Screen use, headaches and migraine

"I have suffered from migraines my entire life. I find when I write more, specifically in my journal or in my gratitude log, I feel better and have less headaches overall."

E. M. Atkinson, The Healthy Writer survey

Migraines can come in many different forms. The headache of migraine is usually one-sided and throbbing. It is often very disabling and there can be nausea, vomiting and problems with bright lights. Sometimes migraines come with an 'aura.' These come in all forms, frequently flashing lights or other visual changes. They come before the headache and can be an opportunity to take medication that will nip a migraine in the bud.

There is a quite a bit of evidence showing that long periods spent watching television increase the risk of migraine and other headaches. Evidence is only now emerging about the effects of modern devices and screens. On first blush, it looks like the findings are going to be much the same. All screens make headaches and migraine worse.

In a study of nearly 5000 French students, it was shown that those who had the highest screen-time use (more than two hours daily) had a 37% increased likelihood of migraine. The results suggest that even the smaller screens carry the same risk as has previously been found with studies of television use. It was noted that non-migraine headaches didn't seem to be increased at all.

Tension and other non-migraine headaches

Tension headaches are often described as feeling like a band or pressure around the head or in the neck region. They can be persistent and last for prolonged periods of time, even days and weeks. They don't tend to cause symptoms like vomiting or the typical 'aura' that people can get with migraine, but some people may feel nauseated with them.

Tension headaches are often related to stress, and it's important to have an awareness of this. In addition, they might be exacerbated by postural problems, and if you are craning over your computer screen, sitting on dodgy coffee shop sofas while you hack away at your laptop, you may be at greater risk. It would not be surprising if you develop some headache symptoms as a result.

The briefest of glances at an anatomical model of muscles will make it very obvious that the neck and the head area has several thick layers of muscle. Some of these are the tiny muscles of facial expression but most are rather more workman-like and extend all around the head as well as down into the neck.

This means that postural problems can result in neck pain and that can very easily become a headache if the muscles affected are those that sit across the forehead and the temple region. Sometimes the muscles will be tender and there may be trigger points in certain places.

Sometimes headaches can also be caused by the overuse of painkilling medications. This is important to bear in mind in the case of persistent headaches without any other obvious cause.

Managing general non-migraine headaches

These kind of headaches are often persistent and do not respond well to pain relief medication.

Often in headaches that are muscular in nature some kind of physical therapy is helpful in settling them down. It may be that the stress associated with your work can be exacerbating these as well. We've all had that feeling of rising stress and our shoulders coming up to meet our ears as we get more and more tense. Simple exercises are often helpful. Getting the ergonomics of your workstation right also matter, which we cover in Part 2.

Getting some kind of general exercise can also make a huge difference. There's nothing like exercise to shake out general muscle tension, reduce stress and anxiety, and promote normal posture.

There are some medications that can be used for people suffering from persistent tension headaches, but these will need to be discussed with your healthcare professional. In the meantime, you should be thinking hard about the amount of time you spend in front of the computer, considering options like dictation and exploring physical treatments such as massage, hot baths, and getting some exercise.

Sometimes, the understanding that these headaches are caused by something which is ultimately non-sinister can make a huge difference. When people have a headache that lasts a couple of weeks, they often think the worst and a diagnosis like brain tumor bubbles up quickly in any con- sultations with Dr Google.

It is worth bearing in mind that tension headaches are ten a penny. Headaches due to brain tumors are rare indeed. A conversation with your healthcare professional to confirm there's nothing more sinister going on can often be enough to settle that anxiety.

Strategies to reduce screen time to help eye strain and headaches

How do we do anything about these problems of eye strain and headaches?

One of the most obvious things to do is **reduce screen-time**.

There are a number of strategies you can try that won't actually stop you from writing. There may be some scope in using pen and paper. Even if it's not something you could consider for the main body of your writing, then you may be able to go analog for short bursts. Some people find this useful for planning and preparing before the actual writing.

Joanna and I both edit drafts on paper before going back to the computer. Dictation also offers a chance to get away from the tyranny of the screen. Almost all strategies will involve regular breaks but there is one important point:

Ensure your breaks actually involve time away from a screen.

It is all too easy to put aside the writing work in progress and then check social media or email on your phone or another browser tab.

You might be refreshing your creative juices ready for another bout of writing, but you are certainly not giving your eyeballs a break. It is common these days to see people scrolling through their phones as they eat their lunch. In fact, there is scarcely a human activity that isn't being done right now by someone while simultaneously looking at a screen. You know it's true. Make sure you actually get away from the screen for your breaks. Close your eyes, look at something else. Go for a walk and gaze into the far distance.

"I suffer from dry eyes, eye strain, and mental screen burnout where I have to go for a trail run or something just to get away from my computer. On a couple occasions, I've had eye strain so bad I have to avoid a computer for a day or two.

Now I regularly use eye drops as well as an app called f.lux to regulate my screen color as I approach bedtime to eliminate the blues, as well as night shift on my iPhone."

John Lilley, The Healthy Writer survey

Managing eyestrain and headaches

Here are some options if you are suffering from eyestrain and headaches.

Keep a diary.

Headache diaries are particularly important, as they can pick up triggers from food, screen use, or other patterns such as cyclical headaches that could be hormonal.

Use a printed page and write down your pain levels per day as well as what else you're doing that might be related e.g. *Headache 5/10 - worked on computer for 4 hours straight. Drank too much coffee.* Once you've done this for 30 days, you should be able to see some patterns.

Think of the pain in layers.

Tackle one thing at a time and see if you can dissolve them away.

For example, if you are an introvert in a high-stimulus working environment, try wearing noise-canceling headphones. If you're working to high-stress deadlines, re-organize your work, negotiate extensions and lessen your stress. Consider talking to your doctor about different forms of medication. Incorporate some of the tips around back pain, diet, and exercise for a more holistic approach.

Blink regularly!

Easier said than done given the unconscious nature of blinking. The best way is to build in regular, structured breaks into your working day. For example, the Pomodoro Method involves working for short periods, often 25 minutes, before taking a short break.

Consider eye drops.

Some people may get benefit from using artificial tears or other simple eye drops when they spend a lot of time working in front of a computer screen.

See an optician.

You might actually need to correct your vision, and if you are running a business as an author, an optician's visit can be a deductible expense as it is critical for the job.

[*Note from Joanna:* I wear contact lenses, which help me to blink more because they dry out faster than eyeballs do! I also found that moving to daily disposables helped a lot with the eye infections that are common if you wear month-long lenses.]

Consider using a blue-light screen filter.

These help to reduce reflection on the glare from the screen and have been shown to help prevent the reduction in blink rate. Studies have shown that there is significantly less eye strain in people who use screen filters.

Sit further away.

Distance to the screen is an important factor in eye strain, and people who sat more than 50cm from their screen had fewer symptoms. For most people that means you need to be at least one arm's length away from the screen. With computers there is usually little reason to be hunched over the screen and it is easy to increase font size or zoom in.

If you are working with a laptop then you may need to consider whether a stand for your laptop, a riser, with an external keyboard is a good answer to give you a better position and keep you back from that screen.

Pay attention to the surrounding light.

One study showed that people who use computers in a very bright or very dark room were more prone to visual symptoms. This is probably due to reflections, and adjustments to your screen brightness and contrast may help reduce symptoms.

Questions:

- Do you suffer from eye strain or headaches? Can you track when this occurs and try to work out whether it relates to screen use?

- When was the last time you went to an optician?

- Would you benefit from getting a screen filter or sitting further away from your computer screen?

Resources:

- The strategies in Part 2 around improving your work space, taking breaks, diet, and exercise will help with these issues.

1.9 A personal story of headache and migraine

Headaches have been a part of my life for as long as I can remember.

I (Joanna) started wearing glasses at age 12, but as a teenager, I rebelled against them and used to go out without them, giving myself significant eye strain for the sake of vanity. I moved to contact lenses at 19, but then spent long hours in the library at university and started at a corporate desk job in 1997. Since then, I have spent the majority of my working life in front of a computer.

I should have taken out shares in big Pharma based on the number of painkillers I took in those days. I popped ibuprofen like candy to keep the headaches at bay while I did my work, most often in large, open-plan offices. At one point, my office was like a high-intensity farm, with hundreds of us in cubicles separated by low-rise dividers. Cubicle slave, indeed! The level of noise and sensation in the room was torture for me as a hyper-sensitive introvert, and this was before the days when wearing headphones was acceptable.

Little tip: if you work in this kind of open-plan environment, invest in some noise-canceling headphones as they make a lot of difference to being able to shut out sound and distraction.

During those corporate days, my headaches were a combination of over-stimulation and work-related stress, plus hours concentrating in front of a screen, plus eye strain, with some added dehydration because of enthusiastic air-conditioning.

I had always experienced hormonal migraines once a month, but they had increased to once a week because of my lifestyle. When the head pain got too much, I ended up in bed in the dark with a cold flannel on my face for hours at a time. I thought that head pain was just part of my life, but it was getting worse as my work-related stress increased. I cried a lot in those days, frustrated and angry. I hated what I was doing with my life, but I was also in pain a lot of the time.

Here's an excerpt from my journal at that time.

"I feel the pinching of my spine and the taut muscles in my neck as the screws tighten. Throbbing curves around my ears and down into my shoulders. Someone has bashed me with a baseball bat at the edge of my skull, smashing the bone into my brain. Two bars of steel bore through my eyes and the surface of my eyeballs expand from pressure.

Light is torture. Pixels split into too much detail and everything is magnified and in capitals. Sound is amplified to a roar made up of billions of tiny noises all crowding for attention. Breathing sounds like a deafening waterfall, a footfall is a crash, music a thudding cacophony. There's buzzing in my ears, an insect trying to get out or blood knocking on my brain. My vision narrows as a mask, pink and orange patches dancing on the walls. My legs wobble as I struggle to get somewhere dark and quiet before I collapse into a wreck of tears."

It was around this time in 2006 that I started writing what would become *Career Change*, a book about finding work we love. I discovered writing, self-publishing, blogging and a whole community of people making their living online. Suddenly, I saw a future where I didn't have to work in such a high-stress environment, and I began working to make that a reality.

You can find the highlights of my journey at www.TheCreativePenn.com/timeline

In 2011, I left that corporate job and my stress headaches disappeared quickly because I removed myself from that high-stimulus environment, stopped doing work I hated and moved away from the stress imposed by all-consuming deadlines and the relentless project life-cycle.

But I still had head pain.

So, perhaps we need to think about pain as multi-leveled

You can soften away one layer, deal with the problem that causes it, only to find another level below.

As authors, it's all too easy to stress ourselves out with deadlines, whether contractual or self-imposed. We work hours in front of the computer, unblinking, chin out like a tortoise, putting strain on our necks and causing tension headaches. Back pain and headaches were tied together for me and as I outlined in Chapter 1.3, I resolved a lot of this over time with changes to my work environment, walking, and yoga.

But I still experienced hormonal migraines, so I went back to the doctor and switched to a different contraceptive pill. It was like a miracle! My monthly migraines disappeared completely. I had been on that same pill for 15 years by the time I changed, and I had assumed that the various side effects were just the same across different medications. But they were completely different. I kicked myself that I hadn't thought about switching earlier.

So am I a completely headache-free zone these days? A paragon of healthy virtue?

Of course not! But because I have removed the biggest reasons for regular headaches and migraine, I am acutely aware of when I cause a headache through my own actions.

My headaches and very occasional migraines these days are generally related to speaking and going to conferences, where the amount of stimulation and noise sends my stress levels soaring. I love that I can change people's lives by speaking and I enjoy the learning experience of conferences, but I pop pills during the events and tend to experience a week of pain afterward. You'll find me in my reading chair with a hot wheat-pack around my neck being very quiet.

There may come a day when I decide that live events are just not worth it, but for now, some form of occasional pain is a trade-off I am willing to make for the positive benefits.

Pain is our body saying that something is wrong.

It's feedback, but only if we listen.

1.10 Loneliness and isolation

"Writing is a lonely job. Even if a writer socializes regularly, when he gets down to the real business of his life, it is he and his typewriter or word processor. No one else is or can be involved in the matter."

Isaac Asimov

There is a romantic notion that a writer needs to be secreted away, locked in their garret, tortured by their creativity, apart from other people. They are special and only need the Muse for company.

And indeed, you do have to sit down on your own and do the writing if you are a writer. There's no getting away from the fundamentally solitary nature of that basic task. You do not spend large amounts of the writer's day job in team meetings, schmoozing clients, trying to persuade people to buy your product or invest in your business. The core of what we do involves sitting (or standing) and occupying the space between our ears.

Of course, many authors do engage in social activities as part of their role, as well as the tasks that are involved in running a business. But little of this may be face-to-face and much of it will be done via the internet and email these days. All authors may be involved in marketing, writers' conferences and conferences, or book signings. These activities are often regarded with a certain amount of trepidation, if not outright horror, by many writers who are deeply introverted. In comparison, extroverts may suffer even more from the solitary nature of writing.

The question is: how much does social isolation affect your health?

The short answer is that it matters a lot.

Most of the research into social isolation has been done in populations that have been particularly prone to the effects, for example, older adults and those with mental health problems.

The medical evidence has been expanding out and looking further into society to see how far the experience of being lonely can affect health. Increasingly, we live in communities that are, ironically, considering our connected world, more isolated than ever before. We may not engage with our neighbors, we won't know the people living in our street or in our town. There may be many more of us on the planet but, in terms of close personal relationships, connections are diminishing in quality. Of course, modern technology plays a large part in this but the impact of social media is only just being realized. We are in its infancy. We're not sure how it's going to affect human relationships and the way we engage with each other in the future.

It is often stated that human beings are naturally social creatures. This seems reasonably self-evident. We tend to gather together and we don't live solitary existences.

"I've had a hard time finding my tribe for the emotional support. And at the end of my writing days (days I dedicate to writing) I feel lonely and off. I still love it and am dedicated but the journey can be rough."

Maryann Jacobsen, The Healthy Writer survey

Loneliness is as bad for your health as smoking

It has been described as an epidemic. Surveys have pointed to increasing concern amongst people that they are lonely, or that their friends are lonely. People think that life in general is lonelier than it used to be, and there is clear evidence of the damaging effects of loneliness on our health.

One study in 2010 gathered together all the reviews on the health effects of loneliness. In total there were 148 studies with over 300,000 people. There was a 50% greater chance of survival in people who had stronger social relationships. This remained remarkably consistent across all ages, between genders, cause of death, follow-up period, and when they adjusted for initial health status.

This puts the influence of social relationships up there as one of the most significant risk factors for death.

It is, in a nutshell, as bad as smoking a pack a day. And, it is considerably worse than not exercising or being overweight. If you were to choose between going to the gym or meeting some friends, there is an argument that socializing might be more important. You could, of course, do both by meeting up for a walk or a run!

Two more recent studies in 2015 performed similar calculations. They looked at actual and perceived social isolation to try to determine the effect on mortality. And they found that the risk of death was increased by 29% in people who were socially isolated. It was increased by 26% in people who were lonely and 32% in people who lived alone. Again these results were repeated across all areas. It didn't matter if you were male or female or where in the world you lived.

This is remarkable evidence.

And, remember, the harmful effect is on a par with smoking. There may be a few tobacco denialists out there hiding in the jungle who think the war is still on but they are few and far between.

So it turns out that sitting isn't the new smoking. Loneliness is the new smoking. As for sitting down and being lonely … that's not a good place for a healthy writer.

Measuring loneliness

How do you know if you're lonely?

Well, I suspect if you asked most people and they gave you a truly honest answer, they could simply tell you. But as with just about anything, researchers have come up with questionnaires to use for their research. One example is the De Jong Gierveld Loneliness Scale. There are just six questions, with three that relate to 'emotional loneliness' (when you don't have an intimate relationship) and three to 'social loneliness' (when you have a limited social network). You can find it online if you're interested in taking the test.

Personality and writing

"One thing I didn't account for working from home was the isolation you feel. It's a major issue and one that needs tackling, and I'm still not sure how to do it. I'm an introvert but I need social interaction, too. You never realize how much you rely on having mindless, everyday chat with other people until it's gone."

Clare Lydon, The Healthy Writer survey

Your personality does matter when it comes to all this. If you are an introvert, then writing is an ideal activity. You are comfortable being alone and spending time in your own head. You may need space and solitude to recharge your batteries. Introverts can find socializing draining and, given the choice, many would rather have a quiet evening talking with a few close friends than partying hard as the center of attention.

It's common for introverts who attend conferences or meetings to find themselves worn out by the effort. Some introverts may use some alcohol to ease their discomfort at these events and, of course, having a glass of wine to oil the social wheels isn't a problem. Having a couple of bottles and injuring yourself while dancing the Macarena might be viewed differently.

Extroverts, on the other hand, may have a much greater need for that personal contact. Sitting and writing may leave them feeling isolated to a greater extent than introverts. Finding a community or arranging regular social meetings with other writers (or related to a completely separate interest) may be even more critical to avoid slipping into isolation and loneliness.

[*Note from Joanna:* If you're unsure about where you are on the personality scale, you can try the Myers Briggs personality test available online. I'm an INFJ, a rare type in the general population, but surprisingly common in writers.]

How being an introvert or extrovert can affect your working environment.

A study published in the Journal of Environmental Psychology in 2001 explored how people were capable of working on a mental task when exposed to quiet and noisy conditions. They analyzed the results according to personality. They found that the extroverts were less annoyed and had better concentration during mental performance in a noisy environment when compared to the introverted subjects.

This confirms previous findings that extroverts are able to tolerate considerably higher levels of stimulation. The introverted subjects were still able to maintain the same accuracy and speed, but it took a lot more effort. They went through significantly more stress to achieve the same result.

Stress is not good for your long-term health and will mean you are at a higher risk of problems such as burnout. This also highlights the nightmare scenario of an open-plan office for your average introvert.

That's not so much of a problem for many writers, but you will want to consider your daily work routine. You may also want to think about whether you find the noise in your local café soothing or stressful. It is easy to tackle with a pair of noise-canceling headphones.

Healthy writers need healthy social connections

If you want to be a healthy writer, then you should spend as much time addressing your social networks and your social isolation as anything else. It needs to be on a par with giving up cigarettes, sorting out your sleep, losing weight, and getting some exercise.

Jumping onto Facebook does not count. In fact, there is mixed evidence about the impact of online social media and its effect on loneliness. One study amongst postgraduate students found that increased use of Facebook was associated with loneliness. More advice on how to find your community is covered in Chapter 2.13.

"The best antidote is to get out and be with other writers in person. Our local writers center offers write-ins, where people just gather to work. There is a huge emotional pay-off from interacting with other writers."

Tracy Line, The Healthy Writer survey

Questions:

- Do you feel lonely or socially isolated? Do you have someone to share with when you feel you want to?

- Do you know your personality type?

- Does your working environment fit with your personality type? Would you benefit from using headphones or do you need a more social working space?

- Do you ever meet other writers? Are you meeting other people at all in your daily life?

Resources:

- *Quiet: The Power of Introverts in a World That Can't Stop Talking* – Susan Cain. The definitive guide to understanding and negotiating a path through the world for an introvert.

- Campaign to end loneliness: www.campaigntoend-loneliness.org

- Look online for downloads and questionnaires related to loneliness like the De Jong Gierveld Loneliness Scale.

- BOSE noise-canceling headphones that Joanna uses when she writes in cafes: www.TheCreativePenn.com/silence

1.11 Weight gain or weight loss

"I've been writing for three years and in that time I've gained a stone in weight. Looking back at my Fitbit stats was startling. It literally started from the moment I started working from home, and it's something I'm taking steps (pardon the pun) to put right by getting out of the house every day for a walk or going to the gym."

Clare Lydon, The Healthy Writer survey

Putting weight into perspective

Just to be clear, this book is about being healthy and feeling physically well.

It is not a weight-loss book and there's no 'fat-shaming' here. But weight gain as part of the writer's life came up over and over again on the survey, so clearly it is a problem for many. My experience as a doctor is that most people are happy to chat about their weight, but no one wants to be judged and stigma is never helpful.

Joanna outlines her personal experience in the next chapter and describes feeling heavy, "sluggish and bloated." Your weight plays a huge part in your physical and mental health, so we need to talk about it here, even though the subject can be a minefield!

How do you tell if you are overweight?

I'm guessing you already know if you are overweight. Most people do.

Some people challenge the assumption that you are automatically labeled as 'unhealthy' if you gain weight or are over your 'ideal' weight. There is a range of normal for body mass index (BMI) but there is an important underlying principle that has to be respected: those ideal weights and BMIs and all those statistics are based on population data. They have taken thousands upon thousands of individuals, smooshed them all into a single homogenous group and averaged out the numbers. So, I agree that it is not automatic. Humans come in all shapes and sizes.

Crucially, BMI doesn't distinguish between the mass you have from fat and the mass you have from muscle. It also doesn't take into account fat distribution. People with more fat around the waist are at greater risk of problems. So, in assessing whether you are overweight, as well as calculating BMI it can be helpful to throw in the waist circumference as well.

Calculate your BMI

To get your BMI you will need your weight and your height. Fire up Google, search 'BMI calculator' and plug in the numbers.

A BMI of less than 18.5 is underweight.

A BMI of 18.5 to 25 is normal.

A BMI of 25 to 30 is overweight, not obese.

A BMI of more than 30 is obese.

A BMI of more than 40 is morbidly obese.

Measure your waist circumference

Take your tape measure and go for approximately half-way between the bottom of your ribs and the top of your hip bone (the iliac crest). These are the recommended values:

Men's waist circumference of less than 94cm (37") is desirable.

Men's waist circumference between 94-102cm (37-40") is high.

Men's waist circumference of more than 102cm (40") is very high.

Women's waist circumference of less than 80cm (31.5") is desirable.

Women's waist circumference between 80-88cm (31.5-35") is high.

Women's waist circumference of more than 88cm (35") is very high.

What should the measurements be?

In the UK, 63% of people have a BMI over 25 and in the USA it is 67%. Australia, a country generally associated with sun and athleticism in the minds of rain-addled Brits has 64% of the population who are overweight by that definition.

There is a cultural relativity that kicks in here as well. The average BMI in most developed countries is now well north of 27. If you have a BMI of 26 then you are likely to be less overweight than the majority of people around you. You are perhaps less likely to feel less pressure to act on it, but you could still be carrying problems with your weight.

My suggestion is simple: weigh yourself and measure your waist circumference.

Write them down somewhere.

If you plan to try to lose some weight then they are going to be critical pieces of data. Even if you don't, I recommend making a note of them. Do it again in a few months. Or at least once a year on a fixed date. Weight gain can be quite insidious. Over the course of six months or a few years, you can find it creeps on and on. You may have no problem with that. But knowing exactly what's happening puts you in control.

"I am currently experiencing some unhealthy weight gain from writing at Starbucks. I have become a little addicted to their delicious sugary drinks. I've been trying to kick the habit but it's one of my favorite places to write and so long as I'm there I tend to have one, two or even three drinks."

Steven Turner, The Healthy Writer survey

What are the reasons for weight gain?

This is a subject of great debate. Many people and the establishment in general take the view that it is down to the long-term effect of an imbalance between energy in and energy out: the old calories in/calories out equation.

There is an alternative view that not all calories are born equal and that the way to tackle the obesity epidemic is to change the quality of our diets. In particular, the view that fat is fundamentally evil is being challenged. The conventional viewpoint is that we eat too much fat and that we should work harder to reduce fats in our diet. The opposing viewpoint tends to take the view that carbohydrates, fructose in particular, are fundamentally evil and they should be eradicated from our diets.

Me? I'm somewhere in the middle.

Call it fence-sitting if you like, but I do think it is important to be in energy balance, that is, matching the calories you take in versus the ones you expend.

I also think that the quality of food that people eat is incredibly important. There *is* too much sugar in our diets, and largely it's dead calories. It doesn't fill us up and we over-consume. The anti-carbs camp also present evidence that this can cause insulin resistance and that leads to type 2 diabetes. If you have a diet that is low in refined sugars, then the calories in/calories out calculation will almost certainly work. There is more on sorting out your diet in Part 2.

It all gets more complicated when we factor in metabolic disorders, but if you are eating a genuinely healthy diet with little processed food, then the energy balance equation does matter. It is deceptively simple, though, because there are a lot of factors that go into changing those two variables. The world we live in and the availability of less healthy foods has a big impact on our eating habits and, ultimately, on our weight.

Living thin in a fat world

"When I started taking my writing seriously, I started gaining weight. Previously, I was always underweight; I seriously couldn't gain it, no matter what I did. Maybe it was coincidence that my writing took a higher priority right around the time I hit my mid-30s, but no matter the cause, the outcome was the same. I gained 45lbs over 5 years. I'm now very overweight."

Nicole, The Healthy Writer survey

The world around is trying to push food at us. We live in an obesogenic environment. And, there is only so much willpower you have in the average day.

The Royal Society for Public Health and the weight-loss company Slimming World published a paper in September 2017 that highlighted the constant up-selling of food. That report suggests that the average person is asked 106 times a year whether they would like to upgrade to a larger meal or drink. They estimated that the same average person was consuming an extra 330 calories per week as a result. Over the course of a year that could be the equivalent of the calories found in 5lb of fat. That is just one aspect of food intake, but it's easy to see how living in this kind of environment puts us under almost constant pressure to over-consume.

Sugar

"Imagine a drug that can intoxicate us, can infuse us with energy, and can do so when taken by mouth. It doesn't have to be injected, smoked, or snorted for us to experience its sublime and soothing effects … Overconsumption of this drug may have long-term side effects, but there are none in the short term—no staggering or dizziness, no slurring of speech, no passing out or drifting away, no heart palpitations or respiratory distress."

Gary Taubes, The Case Against Sugar

It's the demon substance for our times. Go back 20 years and it was saturated fats. There is always something out there in our diets that is trying to kill us. And, there seems little doubt that in developed nations we consume far more refined sugar than can possibly be healthy. And that, for my money, is what we need to look at here: *refined* sugar.

Sugar is a source of calories and it is far too easy to over-consume. Because it tastes good!

Inevitably, that means it has a massive role in promoting obesity, even without the detailed arguments about the mechanism for this. It results in a whole constellation of medical problems, the most obvious one being type 2 diabetes. There are now over 2 million type 2 diabetics in the UK and 29 million in the USA. That's 9.3% of the American population. Even more alarmingly, 1 in 3 in the United States have 'pre-diabetes.' That's 86 million people and 15-30% will develop full-blown type 2 diabetes within 5 years. The simple answer to not developing type 2 diabetes is that you need to consume fewer calories and get more active. I'd add that this is almost impossible to do if you don't cut down on the calories from refined sugars.

In addition, the short-acting nature of sugar often plays havoc with your energy levels.

You get a hit and then you come down again. You feel listless and lackluster, so you give yourself a boost with another little snack. The cycle continues. Joanna describes her experience with this in the following chapter. Like anything, one of the best ways to manage a change in your habits is to monitor exactly what you are doing. Keeping a regular diary, or using an app to chart all your daily intake, even just for a few days, will give you a keen insight into how much of your diet has refined sugars within it.

Weight loss

"I find myself getting so absorbed in writing or working on a project that I'll skip meals or forget to eat, resulting in weight loss that I don't need. The muse is sometimes a demanding taskmaster."

Jamee Thumm, The Healthy Writer survey

This is far less of a concern for most people. Severe stress and anxiety can cause people to lose weight and it is commonly a feature when there is another medical problem.

It can be a symptom that occurs with an overactive thyroid gland or problems when food is not absorbed properly in the gut. Eating disorders like anorexia or bulimia will, of course, usually result in weight loss. While weight gain is generally unlikely to have a medical cause, unintentional weight loss should trigger a visit to your health care professional for assessment.

Questions:

- Are you unhappy with your weight? Would you like to make changes?

- Are you at risk of type 2 diabetes?

- Have you measured your BMI and your waist circumference? Have you written them down or recorded them somewhere? Do you need to consider making changes?

- How much refined sugar do you have in your diet? Could it be affecting how you feel each day?

Resources:

- *The Case Against Sugar* – Gary Taubes

1.12 A letter to sugar

I wrote this while babysitting my cousin's three children for a week. I was late with one of my books so I was stressed. I was out of my usual controlled environment, I wasn't sleeping properly, and I had to do a social event which was stressing me out. I found myself mainlining banana cake and eating handfuls of Haribos (those gummy, sour sweets that are basically 100% sugar.)

I would feel better briefly and then I would crash. As I had my hand back in the packet for the umpteenth time, I realized that this had definitely gone too far, so I wrote the letter below.

Sometimes, we have to hit that point too far in order to change our lives.

* * *

20 May 2017

Dear Sugar,

We're breaking up.

You're an addiction, and you're killing me slowly, sweetly – but killing me nonetheless. I crave you and think about you all the time. When I feel low, I want you, and a few bites of sweetness leave me feeling better.

When I get a headache, you help me to keep working and you help me talk to people when my introversion makes me just want to stay home. I choose you for celebrating, for a treat, for when I need to reward myself for a job well done, for comfort and TV watching after dinner. I choose you when it's sunny and I'm happy, and I choose you when I'm sad, annoyed, frustrated or angry.

You have been my sanctuary for many years.

But you come at a cost.

I hate being an addict. I hate dependence. I hate using you as a crutch. It's not how I want to define myself. I don't want to be thinking about you all the time. I want to eat to live, not live to eat. I want my body to work properly again.

I hate feeling sluggish, bloated, overweight. I hate the headaches that return when I stop filling myself with you. I hate the fact that I shy away from getting naked with my husband. I hate my bloated stomach and the fact I can't fit in my jeans.

I hate waking up feeling heavy and unable to move. The sleep of the insulin coma from the sugar rush the night before. I know that you only return me to the baseline of feeling okay and then when the rush fades, I just want more.

I know that you make me fat inside and out, you give me mood swings, you clog up my blood and lower my immune system. You are linked to dementia and Alzheimer's, and I need this brain for as long as I can happily use it!

You are poison to me, and it's pleasurable poison, but I've had enough.

I can't use you in moderation because I am an addict.

So I choose to be sugar-free. I've weighed up the pros and

cons, and I understand that there are pleasures associated either way, but I'm making a choice for my life and my health, both physical and mental.

I choose to happily say no to sugar, changing my habits so I can enjoy life without dependence and chemical addiction.

Thank you for all the great times, but I'm moving on.

Joanna

* * *

Six months later

Going sugar-free for me was more about overall health, not weight loss. The link between sugar and diabetes as well as Alzheimer's Disease worried me, and I didn't like my addict behavior.

I'm still mostly sugar-free, and I've lost my taste for chocolate and sweets, although the psychological craving still rears its ugly head sometimes. I do have fruit and the occasional dessert at a restaurant, but my taste buds have adapted, so I can taste sweetness so much more clearly now. It's strange, but a carrot or a parsnip can be sweet to me now, whereas before, they were just vegetables.

I saw a hypnotherapist for the first few weeks of giving up. He helped me with the reasons behind my cravings – the need for a reward after working so hard, or finishing something, or starting something, or just because I'd made it to the afternoon!

In terms of my habits, I replaced snacking on sugary stuff with other non-sugar snacks. Little tip. If you want to lose weight, don't use cheese and pork pies as sugar replacements!

So I haven't lost any weight, but I feel better in myself because I'm not bloated. I have more energy that lasts longer – and now I can move onto the next phase of changing my diet slowly.

The improvements have been significant in terms of sleep and mood normalization. I go to sleep more quickly and wake up more easily without that sluggishness that accompanies a sugar coma effect. I don't have the afternoon crashes that I used to and choose nuts to snack on instead of going to get a chocolate bar.

Before I gave up sugar, it felt like it would be the hardest thing I could ever do, but months later, I look back, and it wasn't that hard at all. Give it a month and see what the changes are in your body and your life and you won't look back.

Resources:

- *The Sweet Poison Quit Plan: How to Kick the Sugar Habit and Lose Weight* – David Gillespie

1.13 Digestive issues and IBS

"Our gut is the most amazing giant forest ever, populated by the weirdest of creatures."

Giulia Enders, Gut: The Inside Story of our Body's Most Underrated Organ

The gut is one of the most under-rated and ignored organs in the body. It is 30ft long and the whole of the tube that starts at your lips and ends at your bottom is enveloped in a layer of nerve cells. These specialized cells, known as neurones, are just the same as the ones found in your brain and throughout your nervous system.

In total, there are something like 100 million neurones throughout the gut. That's more than the combined total you will find in the whole of the spinal cord and the peripheral nerves that wind around your body. The gut is not just about grinding up and absorbing all the nutrients you need and disposing of the junk. Your gut has enormous power to influence your mood, your emotions, and even how you think. It has easily earned its nickname as the 'second brain.'

All of this means there is a complex interaction between you and your gut. We've all experienced tummy problems related to stress or anxiety. It might have been an examination at school, a driving test, an important interview for a job, or speaking in public. Chances are that the symptoms you describe will involve the gut. It might be symptoms

symptoms' approach is taken. These
ions that help reduce spasm in the gut,
ves that ease constipation, it could be
dications. These are hugely dependent
is and your immediate discomfort. Your
ave lots of medications to try.

ch with IBS can be useful. Think about
ssible anxiety in your lifestyle and how
ssed.

your diet

have IBS relate their problem to the food
cific individual triggers are often hard to
lactose or gluten intolerance then you will
these in mind. Establishing food intoler-
cky and you may need the help of a dieti-
exclusion diets. Many different diets have
limited success in IBS but there are broad
es that can help some people.

ur 'resistant starches'

not as easy to digest as others. If those foods
ll the way to your colon then they can cause
es can lead to wind and to bloating. Foods
ticularly problematic include:

cessed foods like ready meals, crisps, bis-
eakfast cereals

grains, pulses, sweetcorn

from the upper end of the gastrointestinal tract like nausea or indigestion. Or it could be lower down with stomach gurgling, wind, or even full-on diarrhea.

> "Anyone who suffers from anxiety or depression should remember that an unhappy gut can be the cause of an unhappy mind. Sometimes, the gut has a perfect right to be unhappy, if it is dealing with an undetected food intolerance, for example. We should not always blame depression on the brain or on our life circumstances – there is much more to us than that."
>
> *Giulia Enders,* Gut: The Inside Story of our Body's Most Underrated Organ

Constipation

The sedentary nature of writing can be a factor and being physically inactive can reduce your bowels to glacial speeds. It's not the most glamorous of topics, but it is not just a minor inconvenience; it can be genuinely unpleasant and that's not usually appreciated by people until it is experienced. As well as being plain painful it can be difficult to think of anything else, and it can leave you feeling fatigued as well.

Some medications are notorious. Opiates are a common cause and even the small amounts of codeine found in relatively simple painkillers that can be bought in the pharmacist will often wreak havoc on bowels.

The prevention of constipation is, as most people know, best achieved by keeping up with healthy levels of fruit and vegetables in your diet. Ensuring you get active will help. You also need to pay attention to your hydration, as this can worsen constipation.

If it gets out of hand then you'll probably need to pay a visit to the local pharmacist to get something to help.

> "When I finished my first novel and received the first round of heavy feedback from my editor, it threw me for a loop. I thought I was prepared for harsh criticism; I thought I had braced myself for critique. Instead, it hit me like concrete and I went down – hard. I've always been a picky eater and experience digestive issues related to stress, but this kicked it up to a whole new level."
>
> *Robin C. Farrell, The Healthy Writer survey*

Irritable bowel syndrome (IBS)

There is a risk that IBS becomes a diagnosis of exclusion, left over after all the investigations have been exhausted. And medicine has a lot of investigations that can have nasty side effects.

There are some important tests that need to be done in the initial investigation but you don't necessarily need to have had every test under the sun to make a diagnosis of IBS. You will need to discuss it with a healthcare professional to find a sensible path that balances appropriate assessment while avoiding over-investigation. With that in mind here are some key features of IBS:

Cramping and ab able and they may

Bloating. People uncomfortable.

Diarrhea/constipat these. Some people There might be muc be blood with IBS, It should definitely b cause of blood is her cancer or any other si

General symptoms. feeling tired, fatigued

Options for mar

With IBS you need to given as your gut and y next person. IBS preser and the right way to ma person to person. Here to most people:

Make sure you are **well-h** to have enough water to f result.

Caffeine can be a trigger tling improvements in som cut out caffeine and their b

Often a 'treat th could be medicat it could be laxat anti-diarrheal m on your sympton pharmacist will h

A holistic appro the stress and p this can be addre

Think abou

Most people wh they eat, but sp find. If you have need to eat with ances can be tri cian to manage been tried with dietary princip

Reduce yc

Some foods are manage to get problems. Gas that can be pa

- Any pro cuits, br

- Whole

- Dried pasta (fresh is fine) and pastry

- Bread that has been part-baked such as in pizza bases and garlic bread

Increase your fiber

The Western diet is notoriously poor when it comes to fiber. Most of us don't take enough of any kind. It gets a little more complicated with IBS as it can be helped by fiber, but the trick here is to get the right kind of fiber.

What? There is more than one kind of fiber?

'Fraid so. The fiber that seems to be of benefit to people with IBS is the soluble kind. Insoluble fiber can make IBS worse. Normally insoluble fiber is good to have. It doesn't get broken down in the gut so pulls in water that helps to bulk out stool and that helps the poo get through your gut. That's unhelpful in IBS. Sources of insoluble fiber are the skin and pith of fruit and vegetables, wheat and bran, and whole grains. Examples of soluble fiber (the good stuff in IBS) include oat, barley, nuts and seeds, fruit and vegetables.

The challenge with fiber is that increasing it at all can cause wind and bloating. A cautious approach is usually necessary to test changes.

The FODMAP diet

Joanna gives a lot more information in the next chapter on her personal experience with FODMAP and it is a remarkable success story. She gives details on the specific components of the FODMAP diet.

There is increasing evidence that this can be helpful for many people but one of the biggest barriers is that it is quite a challenging diet. You need to have a decent understanding of the different building blocks that make up food and some of these are quite subtle.

You will need to commit.

That could be really tough if you are eating with your partner (who may have their own dietary needs) and with your family or anyone else. But if you're motivated to reduce your pain, it could be worth trying.

Joanna gives a lot more information in the next chapter on her personal experience with FODMAP and it is a remarkable success story. It is possible that you will need the specialist advice of a dietician to get FODMAP to work for you but it can absolutely be followed by anyone.

Probiotics

There is some evidence of improvement in IBS symptoms with probiotics, but it remains difficult to recommend specific regimes. The research suggests a single probiotic in a low dose for a short period is most likely to be effective.

Other medications

There is evidence that anti-depressant medications can improve symptoms in some people. The ones looked at most carefully are medications like selective serotonin re-uptake inhibitors (SSRIs) and the best known one is fluoxetine (Prozac®).

Some people rail against taking SSRIs for their digestive problems. They suspect the implication is the doctor thinks it's 'all in their head' somehow. That's not the case. Well, it's certainly not what I'm thinking.

There is unquestionably an important link between anxiety and gut symptoms, and we know SSRIs can treat anxiety disorders. In addition, thinking about the gut as a 'second brain' throws the rationale for these drugs into clearer focus. The gut releases chemicals, known as neurotransmitters, in the same way as the brain. Influencing the amount of serotonin in that network of gut neurones helps reduce IBS symptoms in some people in just the same way as it can help the anxiety and depression in the brains in our head.

Hypnotherapy

There's actually some decent evidence that hypnotherapy can be useful for some people with IBS. The biggest challenge might be finding someone that can do it effectively, so look for specific testimonials around IBS for a practitioner.

Questions:

- Do you suffer from any symptoms of IBS? Is it affecting your writing or family life?

- Are you ready to take action to make changes to your diet in order to move toward reducing your pain?

- Have you started a food, mood, pain and exercise diary to track how your body and mind are feeling?

Resources:

- *Gut: The Inside Story of our Body's Most Underrated Organ* – Giulia Enders

- IBS Diet Sheet available at Patient.info website https://patient.info/health/irritable-bowel-syndrome-leaflet/features/ibs-diet-sheet

1.14 A personal journey through IBS with FODMAP

This is a personal story, an anecdote, certainly not a medical recommendation, since everyone is different. But digestive issues are common, and yet not talked about enough because of embarrassment around private bodily functions.

The FODMAP diet changed our life and hopefully, this story will help change you or someone you love who might be suffering from the same issues.

> "The low FODMAP diet is effective for about 70% of people with IBS who try it."
>
> *Kings College, London, information on the low FODMAP diet*

* * *

"We have to do something," I said. "Our marriage can't cope with another year like this."

Jonathan turned his head away, his back and shoulders tense, tears in his eyes. He had been in almost constant pain with Irritable Bowel Syndrome (IBS), and he didn't know how to deal with it. Neither did I.

We had to do something.

I have never experienced IBS, but I am married to Jonathan, who has suffered from it for a long time. This chapter is the outcome of the changes we made after that conversation and the incredible impact that the FODMAP diet has had on both of our lives.

The FODMAP diet has radically changed our lives, and as someone who loves my husband and has seen the suffering IBS causes, I wanted to share the journey in case it can help you or someone you love.

But let's rewind the clock, so you understand how desperate we had become.

In 2014, Jonathan was only having one or two pain-free days a month. His IBS had got worse. Eating hurt. Going to the bathroom hurt. The constant fatigue meant he didn't want to do anything, so mostly we stayed home and at the weekends, he would lie on the couch exhausted. We canceled weekends with friends and family, or I went on my own because he was in so much pain that he couldn't bear to be with people.

IBS is a chronic condition, and I hated myself for being so impatient, but I missed the man I had married, and we weren't having any fun.

One weekend, I booked us a break in Barcelona. Jonathan started on some new medication that week for dampening stomach acid in the hopes it might make a difference. As we stood at the gate waiting to board, he had heart palpitations, clammy sweat and other indicators of heart trouble – side effects of the new drug. He spent the first day and a half in bed getting over the side effects while I toured the romantic city alone.

On another break, we went to the Lake District, and he was so tired and sick that he couldn't leave the house. No walking, no sightseeing, nothing. Just rest.

Relaxation is all well and good, but life cannot be just about rest. Jonathan was 41, but his energy was like someone's twice his age.

He tried going gluten-free a few years ago, but that wasn't enough. The pain didn't stop. We eat unprocessed food. We barely drink. We don't smoke. His anxiety worsened and the pain compounded.

What is IBS, anyway?

Irritable Bowel Syndrome is a functional disorder of the gut. This means that your gut is upset, but no one knows exactly why people get IBS. Tests for more serious conditions can come back negative, so there's no single treatment. Just options to try. The inside of the gut looks normal if you have a scope or a biopsy.

IBS is pretty common, with 1 in 10 people having it at times. But of course, it's not something most people want to talk about, so you may think you're the only one. However, if you start sharing, you'll discover lots of people suffer from it.

The word 'syndrome' is significant, as it implies that this is not going away. You can find ways to handle it but this is you, this is the way your body deals with the world. You have to find ways to live with it happily, be kind to your gut and stay vigilant with what you eat and how you live.

Is there is a test for IBS?

There is no test specifically for IBS, but tests are often done to rule out other more serious conditions, so make sure that you see your doctor and discuss your symptoms. Tests will likely include blood tests for coeliac disease, Crohn's disease, infections and types of cancer – but don't start worrying yet! We went through the whole textbook of awful possibilities, which just made the whole experience doubly bad.

Jonathan went through all of the various tests several times, plus biopsies and scopes. All of them came back negative, and the important bits inside looked healthy. We even saw the pictures. There was nothing technically wrong, so the doctor recommended lifestyle changes.

What are the symptoms of IBS? How does it feel?

We're all different, so the manifestation of symptoms will be also different for everyone. Once again, it's important to see your doctor and have the various tests to rule out something more serious, but here are the symptoms of IBS.

Abdominal pain

This can range from spasms and cramp to almost constant pain. Jonathan's would often be after eating, but also during the night and in the mornings. He would wake up with pain and take Buscopan, an antispasmodic, to relieve the cramps. Some days, the pain would fluctuate, but it was pretty much a low-level constant that spiked at various times.

According to some studies, people with IBS feel more pain in their gut. So whereas I might feel a bit of a tummy ache after eating too much, or something that didn't agree with me, Jonathan would eat something and be in so much pain that he would need to lie down or go to bed or sit on the toilet for a long time. This level of pain leads to anxiety because of the concern that there is something really wrong. Reading about this pain sensitivity has helped a great deal because it lessened his anxiety around pain levels.

Bloating and swelling

Sometimes Jonathan's belly would swell up like a beach ball, and his face would get bloated as well. Sometimes the bloating would be accompanied by a clammy sweat.

Difficulty with bowel function

This might range from diarrhea to constipation, as well as wind and stomach noises. This can also mean a desperate need to get to a toilet quickly and the embarrassment that can accompany any kind of bathroom activity. You find yourself planning journeys around bathroom stops. Stools range in size and consistency.

[Note from Euan: Blood in the stool is not a symptom of IBS and can be serious, so make sure you get this checked out. It can also be from straining too much or hemorrhoids, but it's best to get it checked out with your doctor.]

Nausea

Sometimes Jonathan would feel so bad, he couldn't walk. He just needed to lie down.

There may be other physical symptoms that may include backache, muscle pains, heartburn, and bladder symptoms.

Anxiety

If every meal you eat gives you pain, then anxiety will be pretty much a part of the experience, because you believe there's something horribly wrong, even if the doctor can't find anything on the tests. Believe me, we had a lot of tests and they all came back negative.

Fatigue

A deep exhaustion, not wanting to do anything, sleeping a lot, needing a lot of rest but never getting enough. A general lethargy that prevents much activity. Pain is very tiring and so is anxiety, so the fatigue may be related to those aspects, but it can become so acute that it stops you doing most things.

I've had fatigue at times in my life caused by work burnout and eventually, it would get so bad that I would have to drop everything for a week or two and recover. But fatigue every day for years? That is something more associated with chronic illness and that's what was most affecting our relationship, because we couldn't do much at weekends and every holiday was impacted by his sickness.

Jonathan used a couple of common medicines for the temporary relief of pain, Buscopan and peppermint oil. We used the Colpermin brand but there are others. These are anti-spasmodics, which means that they relax the gut muscles.

He also took water-soluble fiber powder to help with bowel movements. But once Jonathan had spent a couple of weeks on the FODMAP diet, he was able to stop using all these medications as he didn't need them anymore.

Within 48 hours of changing to the FODMAP diet, Jonathan's fatigue lifted.

"For the first time, I know the difference between tired and fatigue," he said. "And I don't have fatigue anymore."

What is FODMAP?

FODMAP is an acronym and stands for:

Fermentable

Oligosaccharides

Disaccharides

Monosaccharides

And

Polyols

These are types of sugars found naturally in different foods and some people with IBS have sensitivities to specific types. The best book to read is *The Complete Low FODMAP Diet* by Dr Sue Shepherd and Dr Peter Gibson. The authors are medical doctors specializing in gut disorders and IBS specifically.

There are also smartphone apps. After trying a few, we found the Monash University Low FODMAP Diet app to be the best. It's the more pricey one, but it is well worth it. The app has traffic lights on foods and you can see which category they fit into. Once you've tested different categories e.g. polyols, you can filter by sensitivity and add personal notes to help you with shopping and cooking.

Here's my journal from the first day of the FODMAP diet.

"First day! I feel so hopeful that this will work and I am desperate for the first week to be over so we can see if there's a reduction in pain.

I've made a chart for us to use as a guide. It has columns for food, symptoms, meditation, pain level and fatigue. We have to fix things so we're taking this seriously. Our aim is 50% pain-free, as that would make a huge difference to our life together, so we have to track it.

We have both bought a great app with a traffic light system so we can check everything out. I'm still confused why some things are good and some not.

Why are green beans OK and snow peas aren't? Why is cauliflower a no-no and broccoli OK?

An orange is OK but an apple is not.

Perhaps this is logical if you know food science and chemistry, but it doesn't make sense to me. After all, we've been taught that all natural ingredients are good, right? But now it turns out that some are OK for IBS sufferers and others are not. These first two months we have to be hard-core and then add things back in over time."

We quickly discovered that onions and garlic were the main issue and these are actually quite common sensitivities. I used them in most things, from roast dinner gravy to flavoring sauces, so I changed my cooking style. After a few days of excluding onions and garlic, Jonathan's pain disappeared. It was literally within a few days. A miracle!

Here's my journal entry just three days later.

"Wow! Things have changed already.

His fatigue is lifting and his whole energy is different. The dark bags under his eyes are fading. He says the pain is more of an echo or a hangover in his gut now, rather than a constant pain. He even did a little dance on the street when we were out walking in happiness at feeling so much better. My husband is (almost) back!

We went out for lunch, which was a little difficult when you realize that onion and garlic is in everything. We settled on steak and plain chips, no sauce on anything, and that was perfect. Today we laughed and talked and he was so pleased, as am I. It's actually like magic and we are cursing the fact that we didn't hear about this or try it before.

We're already plotting how to bring in some of the other foods to test where the sensitivity is, but we're pretty sure it's onion and garlic, which is in the oligos section of the diet."

You might think that you can't live without onions and garlic as they are the basis for most sauces and used in almost every recipe.

But if it's a choice between pain-free and eating them, you'll soon give it up.

You can use garlic-infused oil, because the fructans in garlic are water-soluble, not oil-soluble. So you get the taste of garlic without the pain. We go through a couple of bottles a month now and it's great stuff.

Here's my journal entry two months later.

"We've stopped doing the food diary and halted the pain and fatigue ratings mainly because they have been pretty much zero for the last two months. It's been that dramatic. The fatigue has gone entirely and Jonathan is enjoying his job for the first time in years. He has the energy to throw himself into work, and at the weekends, it's me who needs the lie-in. The energy turnaround has been amazing.

His pain has mostly been zero or one, occasionally a two. It spikes if we inadvertently let garlic or onion into the diet which mainly happens at restaurants where the food isn't entirely controllable. But even then, because he understands the cause, the pain is less because his anxiety is less.

I almost cried the other day because he said, "What would my life have been like if I had discovered this way of eating when I was younger?"

How you can take action

See a medical professional and make sure your pain is not something more serious. Then get a referral to a FODMAP-trained dietician who can help you.

"The low FODMAP diet is quite a complex approach and so it is important that you receive good quality advice about how to follow the different stages …
The diet is effective when FODMAP-trained dieticians provide the dietary advice. A recent evaluation has shown that 76% of patients that had seen a FODMAP-trained dietitian reported improvement in symptoms after being on the diet."

*Kings College, London, information
on the low FODMAP diet*

Clear your schedule so you can focus on your diet and control what you're eating for at least 30 days.

Track what you're eating and rate your pain levels several times a day.

Be very specific and use the exclusion method, adding in other foods as you identify what causes the pain. If you don't track what you're eating, it's hard to measure any changes.

Rate your pain level from 1 to 10, where 10 is seriously bad. Rate your fatigue level from 1 to 10, where 10 is back-to-bed deep exhaustion.

Take this seriously and you could change your life, just by changing what you eat. This diet changed Jonathan's life and my own, so I hope it helps you or those you love.

Resources:

- Monash University FODMAP page: www.monash-fodmap.com. The diet was developed by Monash University researchers specifically to provide relief from Irritable Bowel Syndrome (IBS)

- *The Complete Low FODMAP Diet* – Dr Sue Shepherd and Dr Peter Gibson

1.15 Mood and mental health

"Regarding depression, I think the key is acknowledging it and getting treatment. Talk about it. Not just with other writers, but with family, with readers, with everyone. Mental health issues are health issues."

Stephanie Cain, The Healthy Writer survey

It is difficult to under-sell the widespread nature of mental health problems. It is also difficult to over-emphasize just how much these mental health problems are stigmatized. Many people struggle and it's an ongoing battle to tackle the reticence people have to admit to mental health problems.

There is still a societal legitimacy about diseases such as cancer, diabetes, and heart disease that simply doesn't seem to exist for mental health disorders that are far more common and affect people every day in every way.

This section of the book tries to highlight two common problems that are experienced: depression and anxiety. Of course, there is no substitute for consulting with a health-care professional and receiving full advice on the best way to manage these conditions.

There are many people who experience symptoms of low mood and symptoms of anxiety but who would not be formally diagnosed as having those conditions. Being able to recognize some of these symptoms and how they affect you as a writer will signpost you to some of the best ways to get treatment. This section also suggests some important self-help measures.

Many of these health problems are interlinked. If you have chronic pain from backache or RSI, then you're more likely to experience depressive symptoms. People who are lonely will experience some of the same symptoms and can easily become clinically depressed. Being overweight, using alcohol or other substances, being burned out and lacking resilience and not getting sufficient opportunities to exercise will all have an impact on your mental health.

> "Half of the cure is realizing that you are not alone, that this 'illness' actually exists like any other physical illness; you are not making it up and you are not some self-indulgent, self-obsessed narcissist who's looking for pity or an excuse not to show up at work or school. Find someone who shares your pain."

> *Ruby Wax,* Sane New World: Taming the Mind

What is 'normal' mental health and happiness?

'Happiness' is proving to be something of a growth industry in recent years in the personal development arena. Improving your mood so you feel less low and reducing the amount of anxiety you experience is likely to make you feel happier.

There is very good evidence that people are happiest at certain points in the course of their life. The evidence shows that we are at our most unhappy during our 40s.

Interestingly, this seems to be a fairly consistent finding across many different cultures, and so it can't be put down to particular social factors.

Most people have swings in their mental health as they go through life. Serious life events can buffet us and test our resilience. Sometimes we will roll with the punches and at other times these lead to more serious problems. Even without bereavements and divorces and job losses, we will all have a certain fluctuation in our mental health, and sometimes illness will come out of the blue.

Normal is a very wide range indeed even for those who don't have a big serious diagnosis like bipolar or depression or schizophrenia. Read Joanna's incredibly honest and open account of her own experiences and thoughts on 'normal' in "*Delirium: Thoughts on Mental Health*" in Chapter 1.17.

Depression

This is a topic that flirts with the stereotype of the tortured writer. No one deliberately embraces depression in some self-sacrificing way, but writing can be inextricably bound up with it. In The Healthy Writer survey, many people described how writing kept them going and helped them. In others, writing could be a source of distress, opening up their 'dark side,' leading to stress and anxiety around it.

Depression is common. One in four adults will experience depression at some point in their life and annually around 5% will be affected, so chances are that you or someone you love or know well will experience it at some point.

Typical symptoms of serious depression include low mood and persistent sadness on most days. People who are depressed lose interest in their normal activities, the things that used to bring them pleasure no longer do.

Tiredness and fatigue is a common problem. There can be feelings of worthlessness or guilt. Sleep can be affected in a number of ways. Sometimes people will sleep more than normal but commonly sleep gets worse and early morning waking can be a feature.

Appetite can go both ways as well. It can disappear but many people over-eat. It's very common for people to have difficulty concentrating for any kind of period. Finally, thoughts of self-harm and suicide can bubble up, and this may lead to actual plans or actions.

Most people who swing toward depression will remain at the mild end of the spectrum. Treatment options include medication, self-help cognitive behavioral therapy (CBT) or similar and talking therapies with a counselor or therapist. Sometimes none of these are needed and if there is no concern around self-harm or suicide it can be reasonable to adopt a 'watchful waiting' approach. There is not an inexorable decline and, with time, many people will improve again. Sometimes relatively simple measures can nudge it in the right direction. Perhaps reducing or stopping alcohol and getting a little more exercise can make a difference. Those are good things to do in any case, but for those where things have gone too far there are several different treatments.

Author Dan Holloway has written in the next chapter about his own personal struggles with his mental health and how that has related to his writing. He offers some advice on how to go about your life as a writer and find your own path.

Writing as therapy

"I have chronic depression and can honestly say that **writing for myself has saved my quality of life and kept me breathing**. Learning to live with depression has been the making of me – literally. Writing is now my life and I wouldn't have it any other way, even on days when I'm feeling low."

Jan Hawke from a comment on TheCreativePenn blog

There is a considerable amount of research into the process of writing as therapy. Most writing as therapy is used in a quite specific way. One of those is a gratitude journal.

As discussed at the start of the book, there is evidence for the benefits of writing from the California psychologists Emmon and McCullough. Their experiment in 2003 demonstrated how participants who wrote down five things for which they were grateful had better outcomes. They felt better in themselves and their families also noted that their loved ones were happier in themselves. There is also evidence that using a gratitude journal can reduce anxiety.

"When in pain, on medication or depressed, it can be hard to get going with writing. I've found that if I am kinder to myself, don't stress about it and try to do just a little every now and then, that eventually it starts to flow once more, and that making myself write something, even if it's only a few words, makes me feel so much better!"

Christine J Laurenson, The Healthy Writer survey

Cognitive behavioral therapy (CBT)

Cognitive behavioral therapy explores how our thought patterns change the way we act and our responses to certain stimuli.

For instance, we can get into very negative thought patterns around anxiety and panic. If you have a great fear of going into a crowded space, then your brain will do a very effective job of amplifying those thoughts, imagining the unpleasantness of the experience, and potentially precipitating a panic attack before you even get there. CBT helps you to recognize when you start falling into those patterns and helps you to develop strategies to control them.

CBT is the main psychological treatment for many conditions and it has a strong evidence base showing it is useful in many mental health conditions. It is unquestionably useful in depression, where it has been shown to be as effective as medication, and it's a fundamental pillar of treatment in anxiety problems. It is not the only 'talking therapy,' and others may be more useful depending on the problems you are having.

If you have a diagnosis of these conditions you should be seriously looking into getting some kind of talking therapy. That could range from some simple phone discussions with a counselor to full-on CBT or psychotherapy with a trained psychologist.

There is also a variety of 'self-help CBT.' This follows the same principles but doesn't need face-to-face meetings with a therapist. It can take several forms: sometimes it can be computerized and available online, or it can be a workbook or textbook. It is recommended as an option for the majority of people who present with mild or moderate depression and milder forms of anxiety.

[*Note from Joanna:* I have been through CBT sessions for a specific phobia that prevented me from getting basic health check-ups. The therapy didn't remove the anxiety completely but helped reduce it to a manageable state so I could get on with my life.]

Medication

It would be impossible to give any real details on all of the medication options related to mental health problems. This is definitely something that needs to be discussed with a healthcare professional.

The first-line medications are usually the selective serotonin re-uptake inhibitors (SSRIs). Even if you are considering taking over-the-counter preparations, such as St John's wort, I'd recommend discussing this with your healthcare professional. These supplements can interfere with other medications, and you can discuss other supportive treatments, which can form part of a package of care.

Questions:

- Are you aware of changes in your mental state over time?

- How does your mental health affect your writing?

- Have you been low or anxious? How has this stopped you doing things?

- Do you need to get some help?

- Do you need to speak to someone about your mental health?

Resources:

- www.mind.org.uk. Mind is a UK charity that provides many services for better mental health

- www.nami.org The National Alliance on Mental Illness is a USA charity that has resources for anyone with mental health problems.

- In the USA the National Suicide Prevention Line can be called on 1-800-273-8255 or visit suicideprevention-lifeline.org to get help and find your local center.

- www.samaritans.org In the UK, the Samaritans provide a free confidential 24hr service for anyone who is having mental health problems including people who may be having suicidal thoughts. Call free from the UK on 116 123. They also have centers and are available online.

- www.befrienders.org Befrienders Worldwide provide links to national helplines across the world.

- *Sane New World: Taming the Mind* – Ruby Wax

1.16 Riding the waves: Writing with depression and anxiety

Many writers suffer from depression, anxiety and other mental health issues that impact their writing life. This chapter is written by Dan Holloway, award-winning performance poet, novelist and advocate for mental health issues. Dan has bipolar disorder, which means he goes through cycles of depression, anxiety and manic episodes. Here's how he makes it through the waves.

* * *

Why we need to be wary of writing advice

When I do anything, I want to be the best at it I possibly can be. And that means learning everything there is to learn about it. So when I decided, after finally listening to a lifetime's worth of signals, that I wanted to be a writer, my approach was no different.

What *was* different from, say, my interest in dinosaurs or oceanography or playing bridge, was the way reading the wealth of books and articles people recommended left me feeling.

They left me feeling like I must have got it wrong. That I couldn't be a writer.

Writing was for other people, the ones who could do the things so many of the books and articles told me I had to do in order to succeed.

Advice guides tend to be written for the widest audience possible. And that's fair enough. But for anyone who falls outside that group, the results can be devastating. And that was where I found myself.

I would read that successful writers needed to reach regular daily word counts, for example, and that writers' block was no reason to skip a day (if such a thing even existed, which many claimed it didn't). So on the days when I found myself trapped inside my head, removed from the world by the gray veil of fog that would regularly fall over me, unable to conjure a thought other than "I must stay alive," the despair I already felt because of my illness was compounded by reading that I was just being lazy.

Fortunately, I was aware that I had bipolar disorder and anxiety. I knew that made life both difficult and different. And by the time I decided to become a writer I had developed enough self-confidence to go with that self-awareness. I was able, in moments of clarity, to see that the reason well-meaning advice left me feeling so dispirited was not that I wasn't cut out to be a writer but that I wasn't the audience people were writing for.

No one would tell someone going into hospital for major surgery that they weren't a proper writer if they missed their word count because they were under anesthetic. Yet, for all the progress we have made around mental health, we still find it almost impossible to accept that when we are in the tightest grip of depression we are that person, not the person who needs to "pull themselves together and get organized."

That realization saved my writing life.

The general problem: Normal rules don't apply ... except the ones that do

The problem with most advice for writers is like the problem with GPS navigation. If you're in one place and you want to get some place else that's twenty miles down a major road, your GPS is always going to tell you to head down that road. Even when the road is blocked by a landslip.

It's the same with writing.

We are so used to hearing that the key to writing an 80,000 word novel is writing something every day because for most people that's far and away better advice than "if you can do 6,000 words today go for it and if you can't do anything for a week don't beat yourself up, treat yourself to a coffee and come back when you're ready." So we can end up forgetting that what matters is actually "writing an 80,000 word novel."

"Write something every day" was just the way of getting there. If it's a way that doesn't work for you because you have depression, that's really no big deal.

Find a way that does work.

The only rule that's important is "write 80,000 words and make them the best you can." All the others are conditional. You can change any one of them to suit you.

If mental ill health is blocking the road people are telling you to follow, ignore them. Find another road. The only thing that matters is where you get to. The only thing that's really important about how you got there is that it works for you.

Let me talk you through the main way in which traditional writing advice just didn't match my life and my illness, and how I was able to find other ways to get to where I wanted to be.

My problem: how to be 'consistent'

I have been listening to talks, conferences, and panel events aimed at writers for many years now. I have heard many wonderful authors offer much wonderful advice, but while the names on the program may change, the advice remains remarkably consistent.

Consistency, steadiness, habit. These are the watchwords for a successful writer, however they choose to publish.

But many conditions are cyclical.

And even within those cycles of fog, agitation and, yes, months at a time when life feels normal, there can be times when no two days feel alike. Because of this, the very worst thing we can do, especially in those alluring times when we feel 'well' and can so easily think this will last forever, is to plan for a future that looks the same as the present.

What this means is any activity that relies upon reaching a goal by means of consistent, planned, methodical progress simply won't work. And worse than that – the times at which the plans break down, most usually the depressive episodes, are times when the mind is, because of the illness, overwhelmed by feelings of guilt, worthlessness, and hopelessness.

For me, this caused three problem areas. Each one of them could have ended my writing, but none of them needed to – and, thankfully, none of them has.

(1) I was being set up to fail

All the things I was told made people a good writer were things my illness meant I couldn't do. What many of the advice books missed was the only thing that actually makes you a good writer – producing a fabulously compelling string of words on the page!

(2) The inability to do what everyone around me was doing made me feel even more worthless than the illness already did

And if I ever admitted to my writing friends that I was finding it hard, the classic retort would come back: "We all feel like that." People who say this mean well, but it is such a damaging thing to say. The thing is, when I say I can't put pen to paper, I don't mean I'm finding it tough. I don't mean I need tips to unlock the words. I don't mean I need prompts or – don't even go there – a better plan. I mean I can't. I physically cannot make the words appear. You wouldn't tell someone who couldn't use their legs that we all find it hard to stand up, just because sometimes you're tired and don't feel like it. It's time we stopped making the same gaffes with mental ill health.

(3) I used to read articles about writer's block

There is a school of thought that maintains it doesn't exist. If you drew a Venn Diagram between that school of thought and those authors who advocate high levels of planned super-productive constant writing, you'd find a fair-sized overlap. For them the answer to why it's not happening for people who say it's not happening, boils down (logically, if not in words – though sometimes also in words) to one thing – laziness. And so a person who battles harder to get out of bed and put on a pair of socks every morning than many 'successful' people will do to accumulate that success in a lifetime gets the message again and again that they're being lazy.

Of course, we're not lazy. And we're not worthless. And there is no reason whatever why writing shouldn't be for us. And no, I don't mean, as well-meaning people will sometimes say "We all have different goals. For some people that may be the bestsellers list, for you it might be simply to get your work out there."

There is no reason why we can't achieve what any other writers achieve. We just need to accept that advice written for people who are wired differently from us needs to be read with extreme caution, and find the way that works for us.

The solution I found: Working with the life you have

It's advice we find in almost every other area of living with mental ill health, and our writing lives are no different. You, as they say, are the world expert on you.

Be ready

The thing about an episodic illness is that you don't know when it will come and you don't know when it will clear. That means you need to be prepared so that when the clear moments come you can make full use of them. This poses some practical problems such as not really being able to plan chunks of writing time in advance. Maybe you are able to do something about that (if you freelance, or have a job where you can take holiday at short notice, for example) but maybe you can't.

A problem you can address, though, is 'picking up where you left off.' You need to accept that writing a book might happen in fits and starts with long gaps between the times when words flow. That means there's a risk that when you pick back up you might lose precious time wondering where on Earth you were or re-finding your voice.

I have found I can get around the voice issue by using music – I write characters, or even whole books, listening to the same music on a loop. So when I am ready to come back after a break, I fire up the music and I'm right back in that headspace. You might find that an unusual but consistent location for writing (a coffee shop), or prop (a colored vase, for example) does the same job.

In terms of losing your place, whether you're a plotter or a pantser (I am a pantser in large part because I can't write 'consistently'), what you can do is write appropriate notes to your future self that you, two months down the line, will be able to glance at and say 'Ah yes, that's where I was.' For me, that means scribbling a line for each of my next five chapters at the end of each session. It's useful for me the next day. It's even more useful if 'the next day' is months down the line.

Have more than one project on the go

I find that at various phases of my cycle, and when different conditions are to the fore (be that mania, depression, or anxiety) I am able to write some things but not others.

At my worst, I can't write, and that's fine. But when I am in a milder phase of anxiety, for example, I can't write fiction but I find it quite easy to write non-fiction. Likewise, when I am more depressed, I can follow the mechanics and intricacies of a thriller, but find the world-building of young adult fantasy impossible, and at a similar stage of mania *vice versa*.

So I try always to have something on the boil in each of those areas. That way, when I am able to write, I can work on whatever I am best able to write and be contributing to a long-term goal. I may take longer to get there, but I still get there. And if I tried to do just one thing over the same period of time, I wouldn't have rattled off a three-book series – I'd just have got only a third as much written.

Let the ideas come in from the corner of your eye

When you are unable to write, don't try to write. That's one that really flies in the face of the "just sit there and get words down" advice you'll hear from Stephen King and a whole host of others. But really, if they won't come because of mental health, trying to make them will make the situation a whole lot worse.

So allow yourself to give up on writing and do something else entirely.

One of my hobbies is running ultra-marathons, and when I am unable to write, I go all-out on training. And if I am not well enough to leave the house, as is often the case when my anxiety is at its worst, I watch endless YouTube videos about running and other extreme sports. I forget, sometimes, that I am a writer at all. I certainly don't try to force the words. And as a result, I find they often come back quicker, sneaking in out of the corner of my eye when I'm not looking for them – which brings us back to being prepared.

In short, if you suffer from mental ill health, the most important thing you can do is to accept that your writing life needs to look different from that of the writers you see around you. And different from the one you see advocated in books. You will need to learn not to listen to well-meaning advisers, and you will need to learn to say no to the voice inside your own head saying "no, do it like you're meant to."

You will need to learn to work with the life you have, not the lives other people have. And if you do that, there's no reason why you can't end up in the same place as all those other writers, if that's where you want to be.

* * *

Dan Holloway has performed poetry at the Royal Albert Hall, lectured at the Ashmolean, told fairy tales for Oxford Playhouse, and has written for the Guardian, Spectator and many other places as well as authoring the guide *Self-publish With Integrity*.

He has been working with various organizations on debt and mental health for more than 10 years, most recently speaking at Barclays HQ in Canary Wharf for the launch of the Money and Mental Health Policy Institute's report *Seeing Through the Fog*, and delivering the 2017 University of Oxford Disability lecture. He is the 2016 and 2017 winner of the Creative Thinking World Championship and the 2017 Oxford University Humanities Innovation Challenge.

Dan runs coaching sessions on writing and creative thinking that he has delivered to Prince Charles' household staff and the Cabinet Office's Professional Head of Intelligence Analysis.

More details and a selection of his writing can be found on his website www.rogueinterrobang.com

1.17 Delirium: Thoughts on mental health and suicide

"What if this blackness is just a part of me, not separate? What if it is bound into every atom of my body, making up who I am? When they try to rip it from me, or sedate it, or electroshock it away, the rest of me curls into a desperate ball, because they're destroying all of me. I am every color on the spectrum and black is necessary to highlight the bright yellow, and iridescent green, to enable brilliant turquoise to shine.

Without black, there is no contrast, and without contrast, life is monochrome."

Lyssa's diary, in Delirium by J.F.Penn

The previous chapter written by Dan is fantastic, but what if you don't have a diagnosable condition?

This chapter is an excerpt from my Author's Note at the end of *Delirium*, a crime thriller that delves into the darker side of psychiatric history.

* * *

I believe there is a spectrum of madness in all of us, it's just a matter of degree. We all have moments of craziness, inspired by life situations or through the influence of drugs, illegal or prescribed.

Like many of us, I have caught glimpses of what some would call mental illness in my own life. I share these thoughts honestly, as a mentally well person living happily in society. I hope to demonstrate that the continuum is a slide we all move up and down upon, and perhaps help you reflect on where you sit. Here are some of my experiences:

If I drive at night, I want to steer into oncoming headlights. I have an almost overwhelming attraction, perhaps a compulsion, to smash into them. I have to tighten my hands on the steering wheel to stop my desire to turn into the path of death. For this reason, I don't drive at night unless I really have to.

When my first husband left me, my anger and grief caused me to want to self-harm. I wanted to hurt myself so badly that he would be driven back to me out of guilt. (That was years ago and I am now happily married again!)

I sometimes feel untethered from the world, as if my physical body is nothing and I could just leave it behind. I have moments of detachment where I don't care for anyone. I feel like an alien put on this planet and nothing matters. I look around and it could all disappear and I wouldn't care.

When I write, I sometimes read my words later and I can't remember writing them. I didn't even know I thought those things and I don't know how they arrived on the page.

I have experienced religious conversion, spoken in tongues and I once believed the world to be teeming with angels and demons.

Perhaps I still do.

All these moments have passed over me in waves.

They are seconds in a life of over forty years, and UK statistics show that one in four people will experience some kind of mental health problem in the space of a year. I'm not on any medication and I don't think I'm 'crazy,' whatever that means. I move up and down the spectrum, and I expect to continue doing so during my allotted span.

My biggest fear in terms of mental health is dementia, for my brain to die before my body does.

Fantasy author Terry Pratchett's descent into early-onset Alzheimer's started my investigation into the choice to die when terminally ill. It is a writer's responsibility to think about the hard issues and suicide is certainly a contentious one, even for someone who is on the end of their life path.

I support the charity Dignity In Dying, campaigning to change the law to allow the choice of an assisted death for terminally ill, mentally competent adults, within upfront safeguards. You can read more about it here:

www.DignityInDying.org.uk

* * *

Delirium, a London Psychic crime thriller by J.F.Penn is available in ebook, print, and audiobook editions on all the usual stores. www.JFPenn.com/book/delirium

1.18 Alcohol: The good, the bad and the ugly

"Always remember, that I have taken more out of alcohol than alcohol has taken out of me."

Winston S. Churchill

Creatives have a complicated relationship with alcohol.

There is a popular notion that creativity needs a manic spark to fire the muse into life. Alcohol is held up as essential; a necessity for the greatest creative minds to produce the finest writing. Hemingway is lionized for his drinking, but he struggled with depression and alcoholism before committing suicide. Yet many great writers didn't drink at all. Is there any evidence to offer insight into whether alcohol helps or hurts the creative process?

Step up Arnold Ludwig, a professor of psychiatry in Kentucky, who has explored the relationship between alcohol and heavy drinking creatives. He analyzed biographical information from 34 writers, artists and composers. The results were mixed. Alcohol damaged creative output in more than 75% of the sample. However, in around 9% there seemed to be a direct benefit to drinking. And about half described some indirect way it enhanced their creativity.

So, it is all rather muddled with some creatives falling into both camps. There are some good aspects with alcohol but they go hand-in-hand with the bad points. In other people, the effects of alcohol are just plain ugly.

The Good

The theory of the Ballmer peak is that there is a level where alcohol can actually improve your brain.

Not too drunk. Not too sober.

It is named after the ex-Microsoft CEO Steve Ballmer, a super-successful man renowned for his extroverted behavior. It may all have been a convoluted joke about computer programmers at Ballmer's expense, but it taps into the popular myth. It's likely you have had the experience. The one where you have had a drink or two and your intelligence and insight rise to the level of outrageous genius.

Or maybe it's just me.

Psychologists in Chicago tested this in a lab. They got people to do a specific task, called the RAT, that measures their creative problem-solving ability. They then got the people a bit drunk with vodka and cranberry juice. (And, weirdly, they made them watch the animated film Ratatouille while they did it. Which gives some insight into the sense of humor of psychology researchers.) They found that the moderately intoxicated drinkers were better and quicker at the creative problem-solving task than the sober ones. Those people were more likely to think that their solutions were the results of a moment of sudden insight. Turns out it is not just me.

There's a problem here.

While the creative problem-solving part of your brain may improve, there are a lot of other parts of your brain that aren't working nearly so well. That said, it is a little hard evidence to add to the monstrous truckload of anecdote that creativity is improved with a dash of alcohol.

Other health benefits

The other obvious benefit of alcohol is how it is used in social circumstances. A glass or two of red wine in the evening is an important pleasure in many people's life. A little disinhibition can go a long way to grease the social wheels of the introverted.

The encouraging news for writers is that alcohol could help protect the brain and heart. Drinking small amounts of alcohol can lower the risk of dementia in older women who limit their intake to two glasses of wine per week.

"As an introvert, I use alcohol in social situations to enable me to talk to people. As a writer and a speaker, you have to go to a lot of events.

And introverts are not good at parties.

So in order to be social, I definitely use alcohol to loosen the tongue, and I enjoy having a glass of wine, or a gin and tonic … or three. But I am fully aware of the edge of losing control and I have had my share of horrific hangovers."

Joanna Penn

The Bad

Writing with a hangover is not a lot of fun.

The truth is that the good bits of alcohol versus the bad bits isn't a fair fight. The UK Chief Medical Officer says that there is no safe level of drinking. You may complain that public health doctors are notorious killjoys, but they do have some evidence in their corner.

> "I have so strong a sense of creation, of tomorrow, that I cannot get drunk, knowing I will be less alive, less well, less creative the next day."
>
> *Anaïs Nin*

There is almost no system in the body that isn't affected by alcohol.

Alcohol increases the risk of cancers including breast, stomach and liver cancer. This happens with any drinking. There is no safe level.

In higher amounts, alcohol will raise blood pressure, increasing your risk of a stroke or a heart attack. The liver takes a beating from alcohol. It gathers fat, then over the years it becomes scarred and cirrhotic. Liver failure follows.

Perhaps the most important effect for any creative is its impact on the brain.

Creative problem-solving aside, the long-term damaging effects are clear: slowed reaction times, impaired memory and slurred speech. Long-term changes to the brain cause particular unpleasant dementias.

"I have absolutely no pleasure in the stimulants in which I sometimes so madly indulge. It has not been in the pursuit of pleasure that I have periled life and reputation and reason. It has been the desperate attempt to escape from torturing memories, from a sense of insupportable loneliness and a dread of some strange impending doom."

Edgar Allan Poe

Edgar Allan Poe had some issues. It is perhaps not surprising from someone regarded as a forefather of the crime, horror and sci-fi genres. His experience of alcohol is a common one.

Anne Lamott, author of the fantastic *Bird by Bird*, is a recovered alcoholic. She writes honestly about her experiences and recovery and is a brilliant example of someone who rejected alcohol for creativity based on her sober self. Stephen King in *On Writing* also talks about his recovery from alcohol and drug addiction. He almost lost his family during that time, but managed to give it up, and continues to write bestsellers.

From this perspective, **alcohol steals time and your true self**. Your health as well as your relationships can suffer. You may write things that perhaps you shouldn't share, especially in these days of instant publication through blogs and social networks.

Alcohol has a deeply entrenched association with mental health problems and is linked to self-harm, suicide and psychosis. The initial buzz, the euphoric effect of alcohol, has been a balm for many. People drink to feel better when they are depressed or anxious. Yet alcohol also makes those problems worse. It's a vicious circle.

The Ugly

> "An alcoholic is someone you don't like,
> who drinks as much as you do."
>
> *Dylan Thomas*

Dylan Thomas died of problems related to his alcoholism. Other authors who have battled alcoholism include F. Scott Fitzgerald, Stephen King, Hunter S. Thompson, William Faulkner, Raymond Chandler, and Patricia Highsmith. Stephen King has talked at length about his battle with alcohol addiction. Hemingway and Thompson both committed suicide. Alcohol has an ugly face and it has blighted many lives.

What is an alcoholic?

The term is usually reserved for people that are dependent on alcohol. That means if they stop drinking they become unwell and they get withdrawal symptoms such as shakes and sickness. That's delirium tremens, the 'DTs' and they can be fatal. It is reckoned about 9-10% of people in the UK and USA are dependent on alcohol. If you fall into that category, then you need specialist help.

Strategies

There are no simple answers.

Relationships with alcohol are complex and individual. The single most important step is an honest appraisal of your life and alcohol. Where does it fit with you? On balance, is it a good thing? You may use alcohol in a reasonable way that fits with your life. Perhaps it is not leading to any immediate problems and your long term health risk is minimal. But perhaps you do need to cut down or seek professional help.

Keep a diary

As Peter Drucker said, "what gets measured gets managed." This could be as simple as a note on a calendar. You need to ensure you are counting the units correctly. Many people, doctors included, get this wrong.

When at home, it is very easy to end up drinking enormous glasses of alcohol compared to those served in a bar or restaurant. You need to know the ABV% and the volume of alcohol to calculate this yourself but it is usually not necessary these days. It's on the label and there are many apps that can help.

It is also worth making a note of your feelings around alcohol. What made you drink? Was there peer pressure or were you using it as a treat? Perhaps it was something to relieve the stress of a difficult day at work or some tension in your personal relationships.

You can do this the old-fashioned way in a notebook, but there are also specific apps that allow you to track your alcohol consumption. As well as the bare bones of units consumed, it is also somewhere to keep a record of those triggers and your experiences when you go through an alcohol break.

What are your triggers?

Are you using alcohol as a coping mechanism? Maybe you were feeling low or anxious about something. Many people will use alcohol as a reward, perhaps to celebrate an achievement at work or to commiserate and compensate for a bad day in the office. Identifying these triggers is an important part of developing a healthy approach to alcohol.

Creativity and alcohol

Alcohol causes disinhibition.

This is superficially appealing to anyone involved in a creative process, but the consequences of depression and anxiety can cripple your creative output in the long term. Recognizing that you can still be creative without alcohol may be an important step toward ensuring you have control of your drinking.

Give yourself a break

Have some alcohol-free days.

It is known that we build a tolerance to alcohol. Having abstinent days or weeks will give your body and its cells a chance to recover from the onslaught of always dealing with alcohol and its metabolites. Most importantly, if alcohol-free days are a rarity in your life, they are a chance to experience life and your own creativity without it being framed by alcohol.

Questions:

- How would you describe your use of alcohol? How does it fit within your creative life as a writer?

- Is alcohol taking more out of you than you would like? Is it linked to any health problems you have?

- Do you ever drink as a coping mechanism? Could you find something else to help you cope when you hit these triggers?

- How do you feel about having an alcohol break?

- Do you need to speak to a healthcare professional about your drinking? Do you need help to stop?

Resources:

- Alcoholics Anonymous in USA and Canada www.aa.org

- Alcoholics Anonymous UK National helpline: 0800 9177 650 www.alcoholics-anonymous.org.uk

1.19 Coffee and caffeine

"We want to do a lot of stuff; we're not in great shape.
We didn't get a good night's sleep. We're a little
depressed. Coffee solves all these problems in
one delightful little cup."

Jerry Seinfeld

Few substances have embedded themselves in our consciousness as a productivity tool as much as coffee and caffeine.

There is a considerable amount of evidence about what caffeine can do to your body. It is worth being aware, as it is possible that you're getting more negative effects than benefits, depending on how much you take and your own susceptibility. Don't assume anything.

One thing is certain. We are all drinking more coffee and consuming considerably more caffeine than we did a few years ago.

Coffee has been around for centuries, imbibed by the rich. Starbucks opened their very first store in Seattle in 1971. There are now over 26,000 stores in 70 countries. Their revenue in 2017 was over $21 billion. And that's just Starbucks.

The British Coffee Association reports that 55 million cups of coffee are drunk in the UK every single day. Remarkably, 16% of people who visit coffee shops do so daily. It doesn't specify whether or not they are all writers. Glancing around your average coffee shop, you may wonder.

There is a decent amount of evidence that some people can become psychologically and physiologically dependent on caffeine. That's the very definition of an addiction.

There is also no doubt that caffeine can, at low doses, improve your mood and help you become more alert. However, at higher doses it can have a quite intoxicating effect. Usually that's fine, because people then don't tend to drink any more and the whole thing is self-limiting.

Some people would argue that taking caffeine is more of a deeply entrenched habit rather than a compulsive addiction in the same way as some other substances. It's possible you may even scoff at the notion that caffeine use can be problematic.

The Diagnostic and Statistical Manual lists all the possible mental disorders and it is now in its fifth edition (DSM-5). It recognizes several caffeine use disorders. The first, and one that many people will have had some experience of is caffeine withdrawal. There is also caffeine-induced anxiety disorder, caffeine intoxication, caffeine-induced sleep disorder, and one catch-all term with the spectacularly unimaginative name of "caffeine-related disorder, not otherwise specified." Helpful.

The good news

There is some good news with caffeinated beverages. Or at least some of them.

There is evidence that the antioxidant effect of the poly-phenols in tea and coffee has benefits, although there are mixed results. I've read studies that show a reduced risk of cancer from drinking coffee, but I would always be extremely careful about interpreting studies related to diet, as inevitably they can only show associations. Working out causation is a very different task.

There are also studies that show *coffee* can lengthen the telomeres.

Telomeres are chains of redundant and repetitive DNA that sit at the end of our chromosomes. They shorten as we get older and they are, in effect, a marker of cell biological age. If your telomeres are shorter, you are at greater risk of cancer. However, *caffeine* ingestion from sources other than coffee can shorten the telomeres. I should also point out that having a normal weight, staying clear of smoking and alcohol, and getting regular exercise will do far more to slow the shortening of your telomeres than anything else.

There is other general evidence that coffee drinking is associated with a reduced risk of death.

A large study published in July 2017 enrolled over half a million people in 10 European countries and found overall mortality was lower in men and women. It found that in women there was a reduction in death from circulatory disease and stroke. However it was also noted that there was an increase in deaths from ovarian cancer.

There is clear evidence that taking some caffeine on board can improve performance in sport. There is also little doubt that coffee, or rather caffeine, can increase alertness, given it is a mild central nervous system stimulant. A study back in 1991 suggested that a coffee after lunch could help that dip many of us experience on a daily basis.

"I drink a lot of black coffee and it's something
I don't want to stop. It's probably my only serious vice,
if one could call coffee a vice. I enjoy it and it helps
me be productive."

Joanna Penn

The bad news

It is possible to suffer from caffeine intoxication.

How much caffeine is there in your typical cup of coffee? Amounts typically vary from around 150mg to much greater amounts in your largest cups served in coffee chains. A 250ml can of Red Bull has 80mg of caffeine. A Starbucks grande has 320mg. If you get into your local coffee shop and chug back one of those bad boys, you may well over-cook it a little.

Caffeine intoxication is diagnosed in people that have recent caffeine use, usually in excess of 250 mg, and five or more symptoms from the following list:

- Restlessness

- Excitement

- Nervousness

- Insomnia

- Gastrointestinal disturbance

- Tachycardia (racing heart rate)

- Flushed face

- Diuresis (needing to wee more)

- Muscle twitching

- Rambling flow of thought and speech

- Periods of inexhaustibility

- Psychomotor agitation (various symptoms but usually emotional distress)

I don't know about you but I've easily met these diagnostic criteria.

Caffeine withdrawal

The symptoms of caffeine withdrawal include headache, significant tiredness, difficulty concentrating, and changes to mood including lower mood and irritability. Flu-like symptoms have also been described.

You only have to experience three of these to be officially diagnosed as having caffeine withdrawal in terms of DSM-5. Normally these would happen within 24 hours of stopping caffeine use.

Caffeine and other medical problems

Too much caffeine can cause problems with headaches, but it is also true that *withdrawal* from caffeine can cause problems with headaches. Caffeine is known to trigger migraine, and it has a role in people who have problems with anxiety. I know if I drink more than two cups of coffee my anxiety levels tend to rocket and while I have plenty of neurotic traits, I'm not particularly prone to problems with anxiety. I find it is all driven by the caffeine.

I've also met a lot of patients who have had problems with irritable bowel syndrome triggered by caffeine. It's also very common for people to have bladder and urinary problems that can be traced back to over-consumption of caffeine. Some people are just more sensitive to it.

Overall

> "[Avoid] over-consumption of caffeine, coffee or tea in order to keep going, as opposed to going out and getting some exercise, which achieves the same end result but in a far healthier way."
>
> *Andrew, The Healthy Writer survey*

It is easy to end up taking a lot of caffeine in a day. Every street corner in some quarters seems to offer coffee in all shapes and sizes. A systematic review of the evidence of the adverse effects of caffeine on health looked at literally hundreds and hundreds of papers. The long and short of it is that taking 400mg of caffeine in a day is unlikely to give you any problems.

However this comes with a whole bunch of conditions.

These kinds of studies average everything out across populations. And given there are literally thousands of papers it is averaging it out across hundreds of thousands of patients. However, there are hardly any studies where sleep is not affected by late-night ingestion of caffeine, and headaches have been shown to be associated with caffeine in all sorts of ways.

You, of course, are an individual and your susceptibility is unlikely to be bang on the average for everything.

Perhaps you are the kind of person who is a little bit prone to getting a dicky stomach, or perhaps you are prone to full-blown irritable bowel syndrome with a whole host of gastrointestinal and other symptoms that go along with it. What caffeine does to you won't be reflected in the studies.

Questions:

- How much caffeine are you taking in per day? Would it be useful to keep a diary?

- Have you ever had any side effects from drinking coffee? Could it be worsening anxiety? Do you have any other problems that could be worsened with too much caffeine?

- Are you drinking coffee purely out of habit? Does that second cup of coffee, or the third one, really help you, or could it be making you feel worse?

- Rather than another coffee, would going out or getting some exercise help your productivity some-times?

1.20 Supplements, substances and nootropics

"I don't do drugs. I am drugs."

Salvador Dali

One of the interesting things about modern humankind is that we seem to be hell-bent on altering our minds whenever we can. There is plenty of evidence of the use of substances in prehistoric societies.

It is unlikely that we are suddenly going to stop this well-established habit but we are, at least, in a position to offer improved advice on the potential effects and any potential harms from using various substances. You might have just read our separate chapter on caffeine, given its strong association with writing.

Supplements, vitamins and more

My view is that there is very little evidence that vitamins and other supplements make any substantial difference to outcomes in healthy people. And the important bit to stress here is *healthy* people.

If you are well and not suffering from any particular diseases or other disorders, the chance that taking some kind of vitamin or other supplementation will improve your health is very slim. There's little evidence to suggest benefit. There are a few rare exceptions, for example, the use of folic acid in women before they conceive and in early pregnancy can prevent a certain type of birth defect. (Even that could be argued as correcting a deficiency.)

As ever, the problem with evidence is that it aggregates and averages effects across the entire population. This always leaves scope for individuals to claim astonishing effects and it is entirely possible that this could be the case. I wouldn't deny that, but my own opinion is that when it comes to making decisions about whether or not to take supplements, I would rather follow the evidence than hope I was an outlier.

Cannabis

There is a continual and popular movement to reduce the barriers to access of cannabis. It is now widely available in several US states for use as a medication.

Cannabis comes from the *cannabis sativa* plant and is available as leaf or resin. It is then usually smoked, though it can be taken orally. The primary psychoactive ingredient is tetrahydrocannabinol, and it can result in general relaxation and, to a mild degree, euphoria. It has often been associated with people who want deep thinking and it has sometimes been a drug associated with creativity.

Of course, the relaxation effect is often associated with the 'stoner' stereotype as well. They are not renowned as good role models for the productive writer. Tetrahydrocannabinol has been shown to actually be fairly useful at reducing some symptoms associated with anxiety, and the relaxation effects have been exploited by people who have chronic pain and muscle spasms.

One of the difficulties with cannabis is that while it has beneficial effects, it certainly has some harmful effects as well. That's the same as any drug, any medication, commercially produced or illicit. Taking a substance is always going to be a balance of the harmful effects versus the beneficial effects. In recent times some different strains of cannabis have been cultivated. Some of these are known as 'skunk', and there have been concerns that these are potentially more harmful.

Cannabis and smoking

If you do use cannabis, there are a few concerns I would want to tell you about.

The first is that smoking is bad for your health. Surprise, surprise! And the problem with smoking cannabis is that it tends to be smoked in a slightly different and more harmful way. People generally smoke it without a filter, take deeper drags and hold the smoke in the lungs for longer. They also smoke it right down to the roach, where the smoke is hotter and more damaging to the airways. This is a quite different pattern of smoking to normal cigarettes and has been shown to be substantially more damaging to the lungs and airways.

It is possibly to take cannabis in other ways that don't involve tobacco. Using a vaporizer is the obvious one, and it can also be eaten in some forms. There is also rising interest in cannabis oil which contains cannabidiol and doesn't have the psychoactive effects of tetrahydrocannabinol.

Cannabis and psychosis

Another major concern is related to mental health. While some people who use cannabis get some benefit from its anti-anxiety properties, there have been worries about possible problems with it damaging memory and cognition.

There have been a lot of studies looking at the association between cannabis and psychosis. It is difficult to unpick causation and association. People will often turn to cannabis when they get distressing mental health symptoms because they feel better when they take it. Working out whether people are smoking more cannabis to self-medicate or whether it is causing the problem is tricky.

Overall, the balance of evidence is tilting toward cannabis being a cause of psychosis in susceptible individuals, and this includes adolescents. Younger people are still developing and their brains seem to be particularly vulnerable to this effect from cannabis.

For all that, the argument often thrown back is that cannabis is less dangerous than alcohol. Fair point. But the harms of alcohol are extraordinarily well documented and researched, while cannabis remains an unknown quantity in many respects. There are potential benefits and there are potential harms. As legalization spreads, hopefully there will be more studies.

Educate yourself. And go carefully.

Cognitive enhancement and nootropics

A nootropic is defined as "a substance that enhances cognition and memory and facilitates learning."

Most writers have used caffeine for a boost, so few people can claim no interest in this. Self-styled psychonauts have launched themselves into personal experiments with all manner of drugs to reach elevated states of consciousness.

Steven Kotler and Jamie Wheal's book, *Stealing Fire*, has documented some of the exploits of people in places like California's Silicon Valley as they have pushed these boundaries.

Microdosing hallucinogens and modafinil

Most people will have heard of magic mushrooms and LSD (lysergic acid diethylamide). Magic mushrooms have the active ingredient psilocybin and the peyote cactus plant produces mescaline. LSD, psilocybin and mescaline are psychedelic drugs that cause people to hallucinate and experience an altered perception of the world around them.

The idea of microdosing has risen to prominence with reports that entrepreneurs in Silicon Valley have been using these substances to enhance creativity. By taking smaller doses, perhaps a tenth of the usual dose, there have been reports that they don't cause the 'trips,' the hallucinations, but instead heighten awareness and creativity.

There has been renewed interest in the use of small doses of hallucinogens to treat addictions and other mental health problems like obsessive compulsive disorder and depression. The studies so far have been tiny, little more than pilots that offer some promise.

Probably the best nootropic, or at least the one with some kind of decent evidence, is not a hallucinogen. Modafinil has been popular for years, and a review published in 2015 put together the results of several trials and found there were benefits to planning and decision-making, memory, and creativity. Side effects seem to have been largely trivial, with little evidence of significant harm. In general it is only available on prescription and the USA has stricter legislation around it that restricts its availability.

Weighing the risks versus the benefits

There are risks around the use of nootropics. Access has become easier through the internet and sites like the Silk Road on the Dark Web have provided an online marketplace for all manner of substances. Nootropics provide a tempting shortcut to increased productivity. Who wouldn't like to be a bit smarter and more creative?

By the standards of modern medicine, the studies and evidence around their use is relatively weak and unsubstantiated. In most countries the use of these substances is carefully controlled and you may be breaking the law in accessing them. Whatever your feelings about the liberalization of drug laws, the current situation means that access to these drugs can be problematic, and there is a huge quality control problem. There is no guarantee that the medications you obtain will have reliable dosages in them, and contamination and adulteration are real risks in an unregulated market.

It's worth highlighting that there are plenty of cognitive enhancers out there that have a good evidence base: physical activity, education, mindfulness, social engagement, and quality sleep all have proven benefits without some of the unknowns of the new nootropics.

Questions:

- What is your approach to supplements and substances? Do you take supplements habitually?

- What benefits do you get from using substances? Have you weighed these up against the potential harms? Do you know the risks?

- Could you do more physical activity, education or mindfulness as a cognitive enhancer?

Resources:

- *Stealing Fire: How Silicon Valley, the Navy SEALs, and Maverick Scientists Are Revolutionizing the Way We Live* – Steven Kotler and Jamie Wheal

- *Drugs – Without the Hot Air* – David Nutt

Part Two: The Healthy Writer

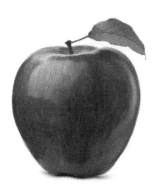

2.1 Improve your work space

"Mix it up. Switch from a PC, to a laptop, to a smartphone, to a tablet, offsetting the pressure on your damaged hands, neck, arms, etc. Go back to pencils and paper. Type up your work when you've recovered or ask someone else do it for you."

Marianne Sciucco, from an article on
RSI written for TheCreativePenn blog

So much of the daily physical pain felt by writers stems from hours hunched over in a chair, bashing the keyboard. If we think of becoming healthy in layers, this might be the first step where you can make some positive changes quickly.

Here are some suggestions that you might want to consider to get your workplace sorted out to be a healthy writer. Many writers in The Healthy Writer survey offered tips and advice that followed these principles, and these are also discussed in this section.

Posture and ergonomic tips and tricks

When discussing RSI in Chapter 1.4, we highlighted how laptops are incredibly bad for your posture. They get it all wrong: the screen is at the wrong height and the angle of your wrists and arms is appallingly bad in ergonomic terms. Getting educated about good ergonomic practice has been shown to help reduce pain and discomfort.

Laptop tips

- Use a riser to bring the laptop up so you are not looking all the way down at it. You could use portable products like StandStand and other options to do this if writing in cafés.

- When possible, use your laptop with an external keyboard.

Check your posture

- Be aware of what the normal shape of your back should be. The rounding off in the lower back is something many people do. Try to practice sitting with a posture where the normal back curves are maintained. A chair with a back support will make a big difference to the time you spend in proper posture.

- Make sure your feet are on the floor or on a foot rest.

- Are your shoulders relaxed? Be aware of what your upper body is doing as well.

- When typing, try to keep your forearms parallel with the floor (at right angles to your body).

- When using the keyboard your wrists should be in a neutral position and they should hover above the keyboard to keep them straight.

- Try to avoid resting your wrists or forearms on the edge of the keyboard or table.

- Position your monitor so that it keeps your neck in

a neutral position. Usually that will mean the top of the computer screen will be at eye level and you are looking slightly down at it.

- Think about your physical writing style. Holding your mouse in a death grip or banging the keyboard with brutal force are not good habits. Relax.

Vary the work you do in a session

- If you can do some first draft work, then some editing, perhaps some dictation, then the variety is helpful.

- If you are reviewing written documents such as paper copies you have edited up, place them in line with your screen and keyboard. You don't want to be moving excessively or twisting around. You can get simple document holders for just a few dollars that hold paperwork up.

Take regular breaks

- I know it is hard when in the flow, but find out what works for you. A couple of minutes every half an hour with a slightly longer break after an hour will help.

- **Do something different in those breaks**. Walk a hundred paces or stretch. Get up and move around. Looking at Facebook or Twitter may give you a rest from the writing work but won't help your body at all.

- There can be a great deal of benefit from taking regular aerobic exercise (the exercise that makes you out of breath rather than pushing weights). It builds core strength, and good muscles equal better posture.

- At the end of it, you could **simply stand up**. Standing and treadmill desks may not be the answer to all your problems, but they do change up your posture. That change may be enough to give your hands, wrists and forearms the chance to settle down again.

"More words while being unhealthy is self-defeating in the long run. You'll damage your wrists, your arms, even your hands if you don't train for it first. And part of that training is teaching yourself how to stop and start the flow so you can take breaks. Breaks are essential to your long term health."

Leah Cutter, The Healthy Professional Writer

Stand-up desks

A systematic review of stand up desks found they had benefits in a number of areas. They weren't quite as good as treadmill desks, but there were clear advantages over sitting down. People who used a stand-up desk burned more calories and people who were overweight burned even more than those who weren't.

Some studies have also found improvements in tiredness and energy levels even after just a few weeks with a sit-stand desk. Participants reported they felt happier and more comfortable, they were energized, more focused and less stressed using the sit-stand desk. There seems to be some evidence that changes in posture are helpful in reducing drowsiness.

However, a 2016 Cochrane review of the evidence around sit-stand desks did not find high-quality evidence of much of an effect. Part of this might be down to motivations. Individuals given a sit-stand desk at work do not necessarily have any desire to change their behavior. That's always going to be key in getting people to do things differently. Certainly, many of the studies around this are small scale. If you are enthusiastic, then you may well get a lot of benefit.

There is also some evidence that people who spend all day standing in their occupation are more likely to get some low back pain. It's probable that a sit-stand desk is going to be best when you use it to mix up and vary your posture throughout the course of the day.

> "I use a tennis ball rolling under the feet regularly to reduce pain and swelling in feet ankles and calves."
>
> *Jade Campbell, The Healthy Writer survey*

Treadmill desk

A treadmill desk is not going to be possible for many people for the simple reason that they don't have the space at home and the cost can be prohibitive. But there has been some interest in this kind of 'active workstation' to counteract the sedentary nature of many jobs.

A systematic review of treadmill desks found that they improved cholesterol and glucose levels. People who used a treadmill desk had reductions in their waist circumference and lower blood pressure. It also helped their mental state and they were in a better mood.

There has also been interest in whether the walking causes reductions in the ability to do maths and reading tasks. Some evidence has suggested that is the case. One study in 2015 did find some reduction in cognitive abilities but the differences were minor. There was a clear reduction in typing speed.

Overall, though, these differences seem to be modest and the gains in terms of activity and reduced sedentary time are likely to outweigh them.

> "My do-it-yourself treadmill desk has been a lifesaver.
> I usually walk in the morning when answering emails
> or doing other mind-numbing tasks."
>
> *Abigail Dunard, The Healthy Writer survey*

Screen filters and light filtering glasses

As discussed earlier in Chapter 1.8, these have been shown to reduce eye strain and will help reduce headaches. Don't forget the eye drops to help keep dry eyes and eye strain at bay. Even if you are working at a café, you can slip some drops into your bag.

Ergonomic keyboards and other devices

There is no clear evidence for these kind of devices, but many people feel they get benefit from their use. Some readers also commented on the use of a left-hand mouse (for those who were right-handed). It can take time to get comfortable but being 'ambi-moustrous' and being able to use a mouse in either hand may help some repetitive strain patterns.

"Ergonomic keyboards for the win. I switched years ago and can't go back. While it takes some getting used to, I haven't had any problems with wrist strain since."

Joe Baird, The Healthy Writer survey

Working on the move

Writing in cafés is popular for writers. It can be beneficial to get out of the house in order to escape chores and family distractions, find a place for dedicated writing, and also to get some social connections. But if you're slumped in a saggy sofa or hunched over at a table that's at the wrong height, you're going to get back pain.

But wherever you're writing, you can still follow some of the basic principles of good ergonomics. Try to be conscious of the normal curvature of the spine, the position of your forearms and wrists, and keeping your feet on the floor. It may still be feasible to use a riser and an external keyboard with your laptop.

"The idea of just wandering off to a café with
a notebook and writing and seeing where that
takes me for awhile is just bliss."

J.K.Rowling, who wrote Harry Potter in cafés

Questions:

- What is wrong with your workspace right now? Consider external assessment if you think it's perfect and you are still getting pain.

- Are there ways your workspace could be improved? Could you make space for a standing desk or even a treadmill desk?

- Are you taking enough breaks? How can you ensure that you are?

Resources:

- Timers for taking breaks: Timeout for the Mac, Workrave.org for PC. Or consider putting your phone timer across the room, or in another room, so you have to get up to turn it off.

2.2 Sort out your sleep

> "Sleep is the single most effective thing we can
> do to reset our brain and body health each day."
>
> *Matthew Walker,* Why We Sleep

Many writers surveyed for this book talked about sleep. There were suggestions for developing routines at the end of the day and recommendations on avoiding screen-time. There was a recognition that depression, anxiety and work-related stress had a big impact on your sleep.

In *Why We Sleep,* Matthew Walker collates studies that show sleeping less than six or seven hours a night can impact your immune system, increase your risk of Alzheimer's Disease, disrupt your blood sugar levels, increase your risk of cardiovascular disease, and contribute to psychiatric conditions including depression and anxiety.

So clearly it's an important topic for writers.

I (Euan) have a work colleague who mercilessly ribs me about how early I go to bed. He knows not to call me after 9pm. I'm already in my 'pre-flight' routine by then, getting settled down.

I turn off my devices early. I get to bed at 10pm or a little after. I read for a variable period until sleepy. Lights off. Roll over. Sleep for eight or nine hours. That's it, same thing every night.

More than anything, I prioritize sleep above almost anything else.

As I have got older, I have got more strict about it. I was never convinced of the logic of staying up all night to revise for an exam, and the evidence shows that it makes you less capable and dulls your brain. If I have a last-minute deadline then I won't toss away sleep for it either.

Sleep is a non-negotiable. It's up there with eating, drinking water and exercising. It is one of the basic building blocks of a healthy resilient life.

Exercise has a beneficial effect on your sleep. If you increase the amount of exercise you do, then you will need more sleep. If I have done a long run or cycle ride then I'll certainly need more. I don't like exercising in the evening as I find the post-exercise buzz can last for several hours and interferes with my bedtime routine. I also need time to make sure I have rehydrated.

"At the end of the day, sleep is a barometer
of your emotional health. And so if you're not in
the right place where you need to be, then you're going
to have voices keeping you up at night because
you have to work through those issues."

Mehmet Oz

There are a few areas that you need to get right if you are going to improve your chances of sleeping well. For many people these will be obvious no-brainers. However, few people necessarily follow through on them all. It has been shown that 30% of people will improve their sleep and manage insomnia by following these suggestions for sleep hygiene. So, if these seem like common sense, then please forgive me, but I won't take anything for granted.

Prepare for sleep

- Stick to a regular bedtime.

- Alternatively, if a regular time doesn't work for you, go to bed when you are sleepy.

- Stop using screens and devices at least one hour before bedtime.

- Consider taking a warm bath in the run-up to the time you would normally go to bed, but be aware that a drop in body temperature is part of the normal physiological process of going to sleep and a bath may cause some people problems.

- Consider a hot milky drink in the run-up to bedtime but this one is bladder-dependent. Some people may be better off avoiding drinks in the hour before they go to sleep to avoid needing to get up to wee.

- Avoid caffeine and other stimulants like nicotine. If you can't sleep, then getting up to have a cup of tea is a guaranteed recipe to stay wide awake.

Make sure your bedroom is conducive for sleep

- Try to ensure the room is dark.

- Don't use your bedroom for anything except sleep and sex

- Take the TV out of the bedroom.

Here are a couple more that I'll toss in from personal experience:

- **Don't sleep with your pets.** As tempting as it is to allow your cats and dogs to sleep on your bed, they will disturb you. Don't do it. (I'm married to a veterinary surgeon so I'm qualified to comment on this.)

- **Get a big enough bed.** Seriously. Buy the biggest bed you can afford that will fit in your bedroom. Shoe-horning two fully grown adults into a normal double bed might be romantic but I will guarantee you'll sleep better if you don't get kicked every time your soulmate rolls over.

There is no right time to go to bed or get up, but if you require or desire a night-time routine then you need to give yourself a chance. And that's it. Most of this is common sense advice that your granny would tell you. Some of the sleep hygiene doesn't always have hard and fast medical advice research that underpins it, but it largely stands up.

Clearly, if you are a hard-core insomniac and have never enjoyed good sleeping patterns then there's every chance you've tried all of these before.

If you are having a temporary problem with your sleep then you may find it beneficial to come back to these and consider whether a few adjustments may be useful.

Consider some routine writing such as a gratitude journal or writing down to-do lists before bedtime. Remember the evidence from studies mentioned at the start of the book.

Psychologists have found that people who completed gratitude tasks slept better.

> "The on/off system for sleep is not like an electrical switch. It is more like a seesaw, with one system pushing you toward sleep and one system pushing you toward wakefulness.
>
> So, you have to be very careful about this balance. The most important thing you can do is to start a few hours before bed to slowly wind the body and mind down. Think of it as slowly tilting the seesaw back to sleep. So, anything that stimulates the mind to wakefulness such as news or internet surfing should be wound down at least two to three hours prior to bed.
>
> Then, it helps to have some sort of sleep ritual prior to bed, which is multi-layered and consistent. For example, you can do some stretches, read, then listen to music. Or you can draw, listen to a podcast. Maybe have a cup of tea, take a bath and meditate. It's a trial and error process to find out what will work and it will not work perfectly every night. But, tipping the seesaw to the right direction is key."

Dr Pranathi Kondapaneni, M.D., M.P.H., Neurosleep Medical Consulting Services

Waking up

Get up at a regular time. The combination of having a regular bedtime and a regular waking time is very powerful. It can take a little while to settle into the routine, but if you have difficulty getting to sleep and then sleep in until early afternoon, it is highly unlikely you will then be able to settle into a bedtime routine at 10pm.

There is no right amount of sleep.

A lot of people are somewhat fixated by the need to get eight hours of sleep. It becomes another area of your life where comparisonitis can kick in, but it just doesn't matter what other people do. Some people need a little less, some people need a little more.

There are also changes as you go through life.

In older people there is a reduction in the amount of time spent in the deeper stages of sleep and they will wake up more often. People are more likely to complain about their sleep and waking early is a common problem. That can then result in daytime sleepiness and napping, which may contribute to problems with sleep at night.

I don't always wake up and spring out of bed with the enthusiasm of a young puppy. Sometimes I am groggy and crotchety. And I would describe myself as a morning person.

I get plenty of sleep, but there is no predicting how I will feel first thing. I go through my morning routine on autopilot and within 30-60 minutes I can feel the fog lifting. Other days I wake up and feel fresh as a daisy. I'm immediately and instantly *alive.* I can't predict it. It is almost certainly related to the point of the sleep cycle when I was woken up.

What I don't do is on the days when I feel a bit narky is to immediately assume that I have had a disastrous night of sleep. That's just life. Sometimes it takes time to get into your day. It reminds me of running. The first 5-10 minutes of a run are often a bad time to judge whether you feel good.

Sometimes it just takes a little time to find your rhythm.

[*Note from Joanna:* When I removed sugar from my diet, especially in the evening, I woke up much more easily and I notice how sluggish I can be if I even have fruit at night now.]

Substances and sleep

"It appears that every man's insomnia is as different from his neighbor's as are their daytime hopes and aspirations."

F. Scott Fitzgerald

My general advice would be to avoid using any substance to help with sleep.

Avoid using alcohol and avoid using sleeping tablets. Avoid using over-the-counter remedies that promote sleep or anti-histamines. Daytime caffeine use could also be having an impact. If you are using caffeine to stay alert all day and then need some medication to get to sleep, it could be that the long-term solution will involve reducing the daytime use of a stimulant.

If necessary, have a chat to your medical practitioner but be aware that the medical profession is responsible for regular prescribing that has resulted in dependence in many people. There's a certain amount of collusion in this process. A patient turns up distressed as they can't sleep. The doctor wants to help. The patient will take anything in order to feel better. The doctor feels obliged to offer medication. A prescription is written. Everybody is happy.

For a short time.

But then, just a few weeks later, the tablets don't work and the patient may have a dependence on sleeping tablets. Not good.

Medication

Melatonin: The prolonged-release version of this has a license for people over 55 and there is evidence to suggest it can improve how quickly you get to sleep and sleep quality. There's not good evidence that it makes any difference in younger people.

Magnesium: Quite a few people in the survey mentioned they were taking magnesium and it had helped with their sleep. There is really no hard evidence for this and that makes it difficult to recommend.

"Get enough sleep! Sleep is the best
(and easiest) creative aphrodisiac."

Debbie Millman

Screens and devices

There is increasing concern about the use of devices with screens and how that impacts on our sleep.

The blue light emitted by screens has been shown to fool the brain into thinking it needs to stay alert. Many devices now offer settings to reduce the effect of this. Apple mobile devices running iOS have run a feature called 'night shift' since 2016. It alters the color temperature of your device and the harsher sleep-damaging blue of the screen is replaced with softer reds and oranges. It's supposed to be kinder on the eyes and apparently kinder on your cerebral regions as well, allowing you to get to sleep when needed.

At least, that's the theory. In practice, there's not a great deal of direct evidence to support that.

Let's be honest. The best way to reduce your exposure to blue light emitted by screens is to put your phone down for 1-2 hours before going to bed. Use the off button. It's that easy.

Like anything, one of the best ways to address this is to keep a log. And, there is of course an app for that. Somewhat ironically, one of the best ways to monitor the use of the device is to use the device itself.

The over-stimulation due to modern life makes it difficult to get good-quality sleep. It is not conducive to good sleep to spend several hours staring at a screen before flicking it off and immediately expecting to be sound asleep.

There is evidence that the act of simply having your phone in the room with you while you sleep will reduce sleep quality. Anyone who has ever gone to bed expecting a call will testify to that.

As a doctor, I've spent many nights on call both in hospital and in the community. My experience was always that when I knew there was a possibility the phone could ring, my sleep was lousy.

"To combat insomnia, I never write in bed and
I make sure to avoid screens an hour before bedtime.
I also get up and go to bed at the same times every day,
which helps tremendously."

Michelle Laurie, The Healthy Writer survey

Questions:

- How many hours of sleep do you get a night? Is it enough for you? Do you feel you need more?

- Do you prioritize sleep?

- What is your sleep routine? Are there ways you can improve it?

- Are you taking any medication for sleep? Do you need to revisit this with a health professional or with ways to improve your practices?

Resources:

- f.lux for Macs is free software that will alter the color temperature of your screen at specified times of the day. www.justgetflux.com. It may help with sleep, it may not. It does give you some rather cool-looking screens and it also has a rather neat Movie mode.

- *Why We Sleep: The New Science of Sleep and Dreams* – Matthew Walker

2.3 Sort out your diet

"Eat food. Not too much. Mostly plants."

Michael Pollan, In Defense of Food:
An Eater's Manifesto

I (Euan) have a problem with eating crisps.

Potato chips if you come from the other side of the Atlantic. I'm a bit of a crispaholic. I'm always wanting to eat more. Even though I am slim I always feel like my weight is wanting to balloon upwards and my natural tendency is for it to go north. It is a daily effort to balance my eating with my exercise and maintain a steady weight but it has become easier as I've adjusted my lifestyle.

Only when I recognized the problems of living in a world that is trying to get me to eat did I wrestle it under control. That doesn't make it easy but if you can build good habits and strategies then it is possible to enjoy your food without the problems of weight gain.

Calories: the long view

Homo sapiens, what we think of as modern humans, have been around for 150,000 years but earlier species that have recognizable human traits stretch back hundreds of thousands of years before that. For almost our entire history we have struggled to feed ourselves. Approximately 11,000 years ago we moved away from being foragers, hunter-gatherers, and turned to methods of agriculture for our food. We have been wildly successful.

We now produce enough food to feed over 7 billion people.

Unfortunately, as you know, it is not equally distributed and some parts of the world die through starvation and malnutrition while others eat themselves to obesity. Yuval Noah Harari, author of *Sapiens*, noted that "modern industrial agriculture might well be the greatest crime in history."

That's clearly hyperbole, and Harari is commenting more on issues around climate change, food safety and other big topics, but there is an important underlying point for us as well.

For a significant number of people, cheap, industrialized food has given us access to calories in a way that was unimaginable to previous generations. The modern food industry has made us calorie-rich beyond the dreams of avarice. And it has given us access to refined food that has profound implications for our health.

It is only in the past 100 years, from the start of the twentieth century, that obesity has become a widespread problem in the population. In our history as humans it is just the merest blink of an eye, but it has quickly established itself as the single biggest risk to our health and well-being.

"It is easier to change a man's religion
than to change his diet."

Margaret Mead

Habits and making the changes

Again, like so many things, much of your diet is born of habit.

You sit in front of a computer and it is highly likely that you already have a routine that involves snacking. If you are the type of writer who likes to frequent cafés, then it is entirely possible that you are consuming considerable quantities of refined sugar through your latte or the pastry goodies on offer. Most of the time, in most people, I would be willing to wager that you order the same thing time in and time out.

One of the concerns of people who are thinking about reducing sugary treats, takeaway meals, and alcohol in their life is that somehow this will result in a paler version of their existence. That these indulgences are what gives life depth and richness.

Somehow, they worry that life isn't worth living without these, often acknowledged, vices. I hear that from smokers a lot.

In the cases of most people who do cut down, who might become abstinent from some or all of these, my experience is that isn't the case. In fact, it is often quite the contrary.

The well-being boost that you get from leveling out your eating habits, from losing a few pounds and feeling lighter on your toes, and from cutting back on an obvious mood depressant, very rarely results in people feeling worse. They always feel better.

Yes, the initial change of habit is hard. It is disruptive. The neural pathways we all have that drive our habits do not like change. That initial period of breaking down a habit, of making lasting changes to our lifestyle, often feels extraordinarily uncomfortable. But, no matter how hard it is, you don't meet many people who make these kind of changes and regret it.

> "By attending Overeaters Anonymous for over 5 years, weighing and measuring my food, and giving up added sugars and refined flour, I have maintained a weight loss of 130 pounds."
>
> *Anon, The Healthy Writer survey*

Weight-loss diets in general

There are problems with weight-loss diets. They can be helpful to shift significant amounts of weight, but the evidence for them does not make particularly pretty reading.

If you are the type of person who has spent their life going on and off diets of various types, then you need to be aware of some of the evidence around 'yo-yo' dieting. The biggest worry is that they don't help people keep the weight off and at some point the pounds go back on again.

The problem is that yo-yo dieting can make you fatter in the long term.

There is fairly good evidence that the effect of restricting calories in intense bursts and then returning to a normal diet results in some metabolic shifts. Our body reacts to this state of semi-starvation by slowing down our metabolism and then layering on as much fat as possible to give us a reserve for the bad times ahead. It is a perfectly logical survival reaction that has worked brilliantly for almost our whole evolution except for the last 100 years for those of us living in calorie-rich environments. There are systematic reviews and many studies that show similar findings.

If you want to lose weight you should not lose hope. But you do need a different strategy.

Rather than adopting a time-limited change you need to make changes that you can sustain. Most people can't stick to extreme weight-loss diets. If you want control of your weight in the long term, your actions need to reflect that. It's not reasonable to go on a faddy diet for a few weeks and expect instant results.

"Cakes are healthy too, you just eat a small slice."

Mary Berry, British baker

A healthy approach to your diet

This is where it gets more controversial.

At present the received wisdom is that fats are bad and you should do everything in your power to cut back on them. Amongst other things it has fueled a drive to put just about everyone onto statins to reduce the risk of heart attacks and strokes. People get very hung up on their cholesterol levels which are, at best, a proxy marker for whether you have a heart attack or stroke, and whether you live or die.

There has been some pushback on this whole approach, particularly when low fat foods are marketed aggressively and people end up substituting sugar into their diet. Sugar has found its way into a staggering amount of our food, including ready meals and savory snacks.

One thing is agreed by just about everyone. There is far too much sugar in our diet. And that has led some people back to diets that are high in fat.

The Mediterranean diet has had quite a bit of attention, as it seems to be cardio-protective. It has found its most recent advocates in a book, *The Pioppi Diet*, by Aseem Malhotra and Donal O'Neill. Pioppi is a small village in southern Italy lying on the Mediterranean coast. If you think of Italy's boot shape, Pioppi lies on the lower shin area. The people there are particularly long-lived and healthy. The Mediterranean diet stems from the agricultural roots of these communities. These are places where fruit accompanies every meal. Lunch and the evening meal consist mostly of vegetables. That's the bit that most people forget and instead focus on the fats.

The Mediterranean diet is high in unsaturated fats but this comes from olive oil (generally raw and not cooked) and fish. The health benefits of fish oils are established and fish makes an ideal replacement for red meat, which is almost completely absent from the diet.

There may be important other factors in the Mediterranean diet that are not all directly about the food such as modest portion sizes, socializing at mealtimes, and the seasonality of the food. It is complicated but the evidence is good: the results of the PREDIMED (Prevención con Dieta Mediterránea) trial showed remarkable reductions in heart attacks and strokes.

If you wanted to make a long-term shift in your eating, the Mediterranean diet is an attractive target.

> "Part of being healthy means determining the diet that actually helps you be healthy. Not the diet that fits with your ideology, or your personal causes, or even your partner's diet …
>
> Think about what foods you're feeding your body. What makes your body feel good? I am not talking about the foods that your mouth finds tasty … I'm talking about the foods that your body feels nurtured by."
>
> *Leah Cutter, The Healthy Professional Writer*

Some strategies to control your diet and manage snacking

This will vary enormously from person to person. There is no one answer, no single solution.

One of the most important initial steps is to realize what you are doing and analyze the daily actions of eating to establish what you do and often *why* you do it.

Work out how your habits are constructed. What are your triggers?

Do you reward yourself with a sugary treat when you hit 1000 words? Do you snack because you get to a sticky bit of the story and you're thinking?

Are you getting bored and losing concentration? Do you habitually reach for a biscuit when you make a cup of tea or coffee, or grab another can of diet soda every writing break? Are thoughts of food just another form of procrastination or, as Steven Pressfield might suggest, Resistance.

Look at your meals

Did you have enough breakfast? Did you have any for that matter? Do you avoid breakfast and then turn up at your favorite coffee shop for a writing session and immediately eat a fatty sugary pastry? There's an easy win there, I'd suggest.

Are you hungry or are you actually thirsty?

Prepare in advance, especially if you are about to hit deadlines

Most people have freezers and you can batch cook days or weeks ahead of time so that you'll always have a healthy option to eat readily available.

Slow cookers can allow food to be prepared on the day (or the previous night) but without dragging you away from your writing desk at fixed times.

Watch your portion control

Using an app that monitors calories, even just for a few days, can be a useful way to reset your understanding of what a normal portion size should look like. Spoiler: it is disappointingly small.

Avoid sugary treats as writing rewards

Try to stick to nuts, seeds, fruit and vegetables. They might need some pre-preparation but you can make that part of your pre-flight writing routine.

Try chewing gum (sugar-free, of course)

Sometimes I clean my teeth in the afternoon when I am really craving something sweet and sugary.

Try not to eat on automatic pilot

Any time you catch yourself eating, you need to ask yourself whether you are having this because you are genuinely hungry and it is time to eat or whether you are doing it purely because that is what you always do. Put a sign on your fridge (or even inside) that will make you think before eating.

Don't drink calories

Sodas and fizzy drinks are a terrible idea but you may need to watch the vanilla lattes. Fruit juices and smoothies can be extraordinarily calorie-dense. Eat the fruit and veg instead and get the fiber too.

Learn to cook some basic dishes

Learn to cook a few simple meals and use them in rotation. If it keeps you out of the takeaway or stops you throwing a ready meal in the microwave, it can make a huge difference to your diet.

Retrain your palate

One of the most challenging things about sugar is that it tastes fabulous. Add in a decent amount of fat, preferably some salt as well, and you have the most scrumptious treats available.

There is nothing wrong with indulging, enjoying our food, luxuriating in fabulously rich and sumptuous food on an occasional basis. Do it every day, do it on automatic pilot, do it without really thinking and you will almost certainly end up over-consuming.

"Make the meal the occasion, don't eat at your desk or writing place. Set the table, turn off or mute tech, no TV dinners. Don't wolf down your food, eat mindfully."

Lesley Galston, The Healthy Writer survey

Questions:

- Are you eating on automatic pilot while writing or during breaks?

- Do you think you could improve your diet?

- Could you reduce the refined sugar in your diet?

- What habits do you have around snacking? What could you change to reduce these?

- How much food do you cook from scratch? Would learning to cook a single dish be a useful step forward to improve your diet?

Resources:

- *The Pioppi Diet* – Aseem Malhotra and Donal O'Neill

- *In Defense of Food: An Eater's Manifesto* – Michael Pollan

2.4 From fat to fit

At the time of writing I (Euan) weigh 163lb or just a shade over 74 kg.

Other than one apocalyptic bout of gastroenteritis in Kathmandu when I was 18, this is the lightest I have ever been in my adult life. My body fat percentage is around 10-11% and my BMI is 22.5. I look fairly lean and I am significantly fitter than the average bod.

But it wasn't always like that.

Before we go any further, I should say that this isn't a tale that will follow me from serious obesity to my completion of some desperate ultra-marathon across the Sahara or through Death Valley. I'm not an obsessive exercise junkie and neither have I ever been sofa-bound with morbid obesity.

I'm just normal.

Athletically, I'm unexceptional. Average at best. I'm never going to win any events. If I turn up to a fell race in my home county of Cumbria, then I'm having a good day if I finish in the top half of the field. In September 2017 I ran a long hill race, the Ring of Steall, in Scotland. I finished in 6hrs 49mins in 261st place out of 440 finishers, so I'm certainly not competing with the elite.

I am occasionally discouraged by this but I remember one of the golden rules when it comes to exercise: *don't compare.*

I get too much pleasure from running. I'm simply thrilled to be healthy and fit enough to be able to do these events at all.

And what I am is Mr. Consistent. I have managed to make exercise a part of my routine and I have used it to improve and enhance my life.

I suspect that's what most people want.

You may wish to train fiercely and run ultras around Mont Blanc or through Costa Rican jungles. You might want to cycle across continents and swim across the Channel. I wish you good luck with it. Follow your heart. Most people don't want that. I don't. I wouldn't have time to write. You don't have to do any of these things for exercise to make your life richer.

So, what do I do now?

I exercise for about five hours per week. I have done that for the past four or five years. Most importantly, my physical activity dovetails with my life. It makes me feel good and it makes me more productive without leaving me fatigued and injury-prone.

It leaves me invigorated without eating into my family time or work life as a doctor and academic. I can play football and run around with my kids. I can run up a flight of stairs or three without any discomfort.

I think I am getting the best possible bang for my buck in terms of health.

Learning to run

I'm lucky in that I have been physically active all my adult life. I don't have any significant injuries or disabilities that prevent me from exercising but I didn't enjoy running at school. I was a weak cross-country runner and endured humiliation in school running events.

I decided to give it another try aged 20. I got a book from the library on marathon training and I followed the program for complete newbies. (This was in the days when the internet was in the process of being invented and going to the library was the way to get any kind of new knowledge.) I started running for seven minutes in the evening. Seven minutes! The program built up to five times per week and within three or four weeks I was able to run a full 20 minutes. I kept going and my tolerance gradually increased but, more importantly, I discovered that running was actually quite enjoyable.

It's mostly a question of learning how to do it.

I didn't go on to run a marathon at that time, but I could run continuously for an hour on a regular basis and, most importantly, found my path to an activity that is superb for maintaining fitness.

In the last 25 years I've had many periods where my running and other exercise have dropped off. I have stopped, started, stopped, restarted. I've been through the process umpteen times as I re-established my fitness then lost it again in a guilty haze.

I think many of you know the feeling.

During all that time my weight was nearly 30lb more than it is now. I just assumed that was my 'natural' weight.

And, indeed, my BMI then was normal at 25. That is still well below the current national average for the UK and the USA. I figured that I was carrying a little bit of muscle and therefore BMI was not fully representative of my state of fitness. And, ultimately, even with a BMI of 25 it meant that I was *below average* compared with the population.

A long hard look in the mirror

Then, around four years ago I realized I was kidding myself.

I had a blind spot.

If I stood in front of a mirror and jumped around, bits wobbled. I had taken up road biking and was coveting some shiny new bikes. I was going to be one of those guys who dropped a small fortune on a carbon fiber bike that weighed a few pounds less, but I was sat on top of it carrying a load of excess weight.

I resolved to lose the same weight and see how much faster that made me.

I looked at my lifestyle and tried to identify the areas where I was taking in too many calories. I know from experience as a doctor that very few people will tell you that their diet is anything other than quite good. Mine was quite good.

Honest.

I didn't have a big problem with my meals. They almost all tended to be home-cooked with minimal, if any, meat and plenty of vegetables. I also didn't have a problem with alcohol. I will go weeks, if not months between alcoholic drinks. The last crate of beer I brought back from a holiday to France I threw out because it was out of date.

I realized my problem was lunch and snacking in between meals. I had a problem with eating while I was in the car. I had a 30-minute commute each way and it was usual for me to eat a snack during those trips. I couldn't pass a newsagent or eat lunch without having a packet of crisps. So, I bought sugar-free chewing gum for the car and I started making a packed lunch daily.

Those two small changes were transformational.

In addition, I slightly increased my exercise and made sure that I was getting some exercise during the week with a specific goal for the overall number of hours I wanted to achieve during that week.

In August 2012, I found the weight started to come off. It wasn't until early 2014 that it leveled off. It took me 18 months to lose 20-25lb.

It took me *months* to lose weight through lifestyle changes I could sustain.

My weight has been consistently lower now for the past four years. The health benefits are significant. I stopped getting any kind of indigestion and I was able to stop taking medication. I get less back pain, though that is definitely something that still bothers me. I felt fitter, I *was* fitter and I got significantly fewer twinges in my knees after any prolonged running. In short, all the little niggles that I could have put down to middle age, to hitting 40, and simply accepted as an inevitable part of aging, stopped.

As for the road bike, well, I never bought it. I realized I didn't need it to enjoy exercise. My old bike was just as good for that.

A work in progress …

My own weight loss and exercise patterns illustrate the time scale needed to make lasting changes. You need to build habits and make small changes that you can stick with for months on end. I never felt like I was dieting but it was still hard at times.

Like with anything, I'm still learning, still trying to improve. I'm very aware that my flexibility is deteriorating and my strength, too. It's something I aim to bring in slowly over the next year or two, but I'm happy with where I am. I wouldn't have time for writing otherwise. It's all a balance.

2.5 Sort out your back

If you get a sudden bout of back pain then you should know that in almost everyone it will calm down and improve with time.

We also know that back pain frequently comes back again.

Many people get stuck in this cycle where back pain is never far away but the slight improvements stop them from taking action. There are many treatments for back pain but there is a lot you can do when you are not in pain to reduce the risk of problems. Building a strong and resilient back is a great investment in your future quality of life.

Treatments for back pain

It is estimated that there are over 200 treatment options available to treat low back pain and there is no single one which is clearly better than another. That emphasizes nicely the scale of the challenge in finding an effective treatment if you're suffering from back pain. On the plus side, it does give you plenty of options to try.

It is worth pointing out that despite a ton of research, much of the medical literature is characterized by a lack of evidence. Sometimes there are studies, but they show little effect and sometimes areas we would like to look into have been little researched.

The other difficulty about low back pain is that it is a condition that needs types of treatments that go beyond pills, and those are difficult to research.

Unquestionably, when I see somebody who is in sudden and severe pain, then pain relief medication can help reduce muscle spasm and give relief. However, the evidence for any medication in back pain has weakened in recent years. When it comes to longer-term pain, then the best treatments certainly include the physical therapies. Education about back care has been shown in many studies to be an important element of any long-term strategy toward a healthy back.

"Therapeutic massage helped me more than physical therapy. Going to the gym, yoga and trigger point release. Trying to avoid the chiropractor because adjustments sometimes make the problem chronic (e.g. over-stretching ligaments)."

Gabrielle Garbin, The Healthy Writer survey

Medications in low back pain

My general advice is to go for the simplest medication, with the fewest side effects, that gives you some relief.

That might seem obvious, a principle to which all pre-scribing should be held, but it is surprising how this basic idea around medication is often ignored. The bottom line is that few medications make a lot of difference to long-term back pain. There is some evidence that non-steroidal anti-inflammatory (NSAID) drugs can be helpful but it is surprisingly weak. NSAIDs also have a long list of side effects, some of them serious, and if you use them on anything other than an occasional basis, it's worth chatting to a healthcare professional.

There has been recent evidence that the use of paracetamol (acetaminophen in the USA), which has the advantage of having very minimal side effects, may not be that helpful.

It is probably worth a tilt, but make sure you take a proper dose. Don't just pop one every day or two and curse it for not working. Take it regularly for a few days and if you don't feel it is making a difference, sack it off. A great deal of care should be taken with opioid medications for any long-term back pain, and the increasing use of opioids in North America has been called an epidemic. There is more in Chapter 1.5 on chronic pain.

Yoga and back pain

There has been a flurry of reviews around the benefits of yoga in the last few years. A systematic review in 2017 found the evidence points toward benefits at three months, six months and one year. The overall clinical effects were modest but were there. It is certainly worth a look and Joanna's experience of yoga, documented in the next chapter, has been nothing short of transformative.

> "I have found Pilates to be excellent for my core strength, and it's suitable for people who have existing injuries/weaknesses."
>
> *Sandy Vaile, The Healthy Writer survey*

Walking and back pain

One activity that most people can do is walking. A systematic review of walking published in the journal *Clinical Rehabilitation* found that walking was as effective as other non-drug methods of managing low back pain. It was noted that one study found 'normal' walking to be superior to treadmill walking.

One nifty study in the *European Spine Journal* found that increasing your walking steps reduced neck pain in people who didn't start with problems. Those that increased their daily walking steps by 1000 had a 14% reduced risk of neck pain. It didn't seem to have any direct impact on low back pain, though.

Alexander technique

The Alexander technique is often described as a method to help people go about their daily lives with less muscular tension. You need to learn the Alexander technique from a qualified practitioner and it tends to be a one-on-one learning process.

A systematic review in 2012 suggested there was some evidence for the effectiveness of the Alexander technique for long-term back pain. The other effects on things like respiratory function and posture were not terribly conclusive.

Interestingly, the Alexander technique has been investigated in musicians and it has been suggested that it could improve performance anxiety. If you suffer from quite a bit of chronic back pain and you are doing a fair bit of public speaking, neither of which would be unusual in a writer, the Alexander technique may be a particularly useful option to consider.

Pilates and getting active can help back pain

Pilates was developed in the early twentieth century by Joseph Pilates from Monchengladbach in Germany. He called his system *contrology* and he would be astonished at how far his program of exercises has spread. There are now millions of practitioners worldwide.

Pilates is a general physical and mental conditioning program and there is a strong emphasis on core stability and flexibility that can reduce pain and improve functioning if you are having chronic low back pain.

The research backs it up as well. Studies show that Pilates can give significant improvements in pain and functional ability in the shorter term compared to usual care and physical activity.

Does it have to be Pilates, or can participation in any sport or other leisure physical activity reduce the risk of back pain? A systematic review found that leisure time physical activity may reduce the risk of chronic back pain by 11 to 16%. That's not a huge amount, but highlights the importance of doing something active.

Exercise is good for your back.

It can take many forms, such as walking, yoga, Pilates, or any sport. Being active will also help you manage your weight, which is a known factor that makes back pain more likely. There is no single method that is clearly better than another, and being active doing *something* is almost certainly more important than what you do.

> "Healing came from a chiropractor visit and advice in readjusting my laptop and chair."
>
> *Traveller, The Healthy Writer survey*

Chiropractors and back-crackers: the art of manipulation

One treatment that is often considered for back pain is some manipulation on your spine.

Doubtless you will have been told tales of colleagues or friends who have visited some practitioner, been pulled in one direction or another, possibly involving a dramatic crack, and walked out cured. This kind of treatment usually comes under the category of manipulative therapy, and it does have a little bit of a controversial past in that it is often administered by chiropractors and osteopaths.

Both of these groups have had some challenges in being accepted in the mainstream, not least because some, though not all, practitioners have rejected the main theories of medical practice and science, and have made dramatic claims for the ability of spinal manipulation to cure all manner of diseases.

In terms of back pain, a recent review of this treatment suggested that the overall size of the benefit from spinal manipulations seems at best small.

Of course, when you look at studies, there may be some patients who get a dramatic improvement, but these are mixed with those who get only a very minor benefit or none at all. If you are one of those who have had your back cracked and then walked out like a new person, then you may well be evangelical about the treatment. The use of chiropractors is very common in the USA but relatively rare in other parts of the world. There has been some concern about the safety of manipulative therapy. There are certainly rare case reports of serious complications where the spinal cord has been damaged.

However, none of the large studies that have been reviewed have identified any serious complications. Contrast that with the well-known and serious kidney and gut side effects of medications like the non-steroidal anti-inflammatory drugs and, in reality, the risks of something like manipulative therapy pale into comparison.

It is important to highlight that while manipulative therapy from practitioners such as chiropractors does not appear to be any worse than the other treatments for back pain, there is no reasonable evidence to support its use as a treatment for diseases such as diabetes, heart failure, or thyroid disease. Issues of physical manipulation aside, one of the things a chiropractor can do is educate you around back care and good habits.

Questions:

- Are you getting back pain that it is interfering with your daily life? What are you doing to improve it?

- Do you feel comfortable that you know enough about good back care?

- What changes have you made to your work space to help your back?

- Could you do more to improve the ergonomics when you use a computer?

- How could you get more active to improve the health of your back?

Resources:

- *The Back Sufferer's Bible* – Sarah Key. Also resources at www.simplebackpain.com

2.6 Lessons learned about writing from yoga

"It is health that is the real wealth and not
pieces of gold and silver."

Mahatma Gandhi

After trying and failing to adopt yoga into my life over many years, I (Joanna) have just reached my one-year anniversary of a regular yoga practice.

I've been going to a yoga school three times a week, and although I started out in the gentle (remedial) class, I now go to the more active classes. My back pain has almost completely disappeared, my functional movement has improved, and it is my sanctuary for mental headspace to breathe and meditate. It's become an integral part of my life, and I've turned into a yoga evangelist!

Here's what I've learned about yoga and how it relates to writing.

No judgment. No comparisons.

As I mentioned in Chapter 1.3, I don't look like an Instagram yogi with perfect muscle tone and incredible posture. I have curves and hips and bumps, and I struggle with body image like pretty much everyone else. But yoga has taught me a lot about accepting and even loving my body, as well as honoring it through the practice.

Just as there are different writing styles, different yoga poses suit different people. There are as many stories in the world as there are physical bodies. So if you can't touch your heels to the floor in downward dog, it's not a problem. If you struggle to sit cross-legged, no worries, use a block or two.

There is no point in comparing myself to someone who has been doing yoga for 20 years, whose body type is completely different to mine, who has practiced those poses for thousands of hours.

In the same way, there's no point comparing myself to Stephen King, who has been writing for nearly 50 years and written millions of words. I can only be who I am and improve over time as I write more and practice more.

Yoga is a practice like writing is a practice

You don't start off doing a headstand on day one of yoga like you can't decide to 'be an author' and dash off a best-selling manuscript in week one. These things take time and preparation and learning and practice. You don't go from zero to amazing in one fell swoop.

The practices of yoga and writing can both sustain you for the rest of your life. I see myself writing until I die, like the late P.D.James, who was still working on a manuscript when she died at age 94. Yoga is designed as a physical practice of longevity, and in India, you see old people doing it every morning as we would drink our morning coffee. I'm determined to be a wrinkled old writing yogi!

Know thyself

Yoga is a physical practice, but it's also about observation of your body, your breath, and your thoughts.

Realizing where and why you hold pain in certain parts of your body at different times can make you more mindful of what you need to look after and help you get some perspective.

Taking time to breathe helps just about everything

Every yoga class ends with *savasana*, where you lie on your back, eyes closed, as you breathe and connect with the ground beneath you. If the practice has been tough, that time is well-earned relaxation, and if you're stressed and manic, that time is much-needed meditation. Sometimes the time drags on, sometimes it flies by, and you want to stay there on the mat, a haven from the world.

When I first started, I was agitated by this part of the class. I wanted to get on with my To Do list. I'd done my exercise, now I needed to get back to work. Lying around was a waste of time.

If you know what I mean, then you need this too!

Savasana gives me time where I do nothing but breathe. It's helped me realize that breathing is something I've struggled with. When I write, I often hold my breath or shallow breathe into my chest. Through yoga, I'm learning different forms of breathing and ways to connect my mind to my body.

If you want to give yoga a try, here are some practical tips.

Find a dedicated yoga school

I failed before because I went to classes at gyms where the yoga class was just an add-on and the teachers did multiple other classes. If you go to a specific yoga school, they will offer many different yoga classes, so you can find the right one for you, depending on your level of pain and movement.

If you are concerned about expense, because yoga classes are not usually cheap, then weigh up the prevention now versus the potential medical costs later. Or check out some videos on YouTube or Instagram.

Find a teacher you resonate with

There are many different kinds of yoga teacher, from the uber-spiritual, chanting headstand guru to the anatomy expert with a sense of humor yogi. They will do different classes and it's worth trying a few to find someone you resonate with.

Give it a month or two, especially if you feel like giving up

I was so angry the first few months doing regular classes. I couldn't even sit cross-legged, and downward dog hurt my wrists. The practice hurt me more than it seemed to help initially and I felt inadequate next to some of the Instagram-ready yoga-babes.

But once I settled into the classes and got used to the movements, I learned how to relax more and breathe and started to enjoy it.

Within a few months, my pain lessened and then disappeared. It has been life-changing and soul-sustaining for me in the same way as developing a writing practice.

Happy yoga writing if you're ready to try it!

2.7 How to use dictation for a healthier writing life

The word 'writing' has become associated with hitting keys on a keyboard to make letters appear on a screen or inscribing by hand onto paper. But the end result is a mode of communication from one brain to another through the medium of words. Those words can be generated by your voice, just as people can 'read' by listening to an audiobook.

Famous authors who have written with dictation include diverse creatives John Milton (Paradise Lost), Dan Brown, Henry James, Barbara Cartland and Winston Churchill. When Terry Pratchett, fantasy author of the Discworld series, developed Alzheimer's Disease, he found he couldn't write anymore, so he moved to dictation in his final years.

So clearly, dictation is a method that can work for many writers and it has become an emerging trend for authors these days as technology makes it easier and faster.

So, why dictate?

Health reasons

You can dictate standing up or while walking, or lying in bed with injuries, or if pain stops you typing.

I started using dictation when I had RSI and used it to write the first drafts of *Destroyer of Worlds* and also *Map of Shadows*, plus some chapters for this book, which I dictated while walking along the canal towpath. Dictation can help alleviate or prevent pain right now, but learning how to write with dictation can also future-proof your living as a writer in case of problems later.

Writing speed and stamina

Dictation is faster at getting words on the page than typing, especially if you are not self-censoring.

I've made it up to around 5000 words per hour with dictation, while I only manage around 1500 words per hour typing. There is a trade-off with 'finished' words as you will have to at least lightly edit to correct transcription issues, but if you want to get that first draft done faster, then dictation can be the most effective way.

Increased creativity

Some writers have a problem with perfectionism and the critical voice in a first draft. They struggle to finish a book because they are constantly editing what they have written. If you dictate, you can bypass this critical voice, get the first draft done and then edit it later.

What's stopping you dictating?

There are a number of reasons why people resist dictation. I know them all because I've been through this journey several times!

The most common are:

- "I'm used to typing. I don't have the right kind of brain for dictation."

- "I don't want to say the punctuation out loud. It will disrupt my flow."

- "I write in public so I can't dictate."

- "I have a difficult accent which will make it impossible."

- "I write fantasy books with weird names which won't work."

- "I don't know how to set it up technically."

- "I can't spare the time to learn how to dictate."

Here's what I wrote in my journal on the first day I tried dictation before I'd actually even started.

"I'm very self-conscious. I'm worried that I won't be able to find the words. I'm so used to typing and creating through my fingers that doing it with my voice feels strange.

But I learned to type with my fingers, so why can't I learned to type with my words? I just have to practice. Something will shift in my mind at some point, and it will just work. This should make me a healthier author, and also someone who writes faster.

Authors who use dictation are writing incredibly fast. That's what I want. I want to write stories faster as I have so many in my mind that I want to get into the world."

Here are thoughts from my journal *after* the first session:

"It felt like the words were really bad and the story clunky and poor. But actually, when the transcription was done and I edited it, it really wasn't as bad as I thought it would be. A classic case of critical voice.

I need to ignore this when I'm dictating. I definitely need to plan the scene more before I speak it, which will save time overall in both dictation and editing.

I did think I would find the punctuation difficult, but that has also been easier than I thought. There are only a few commands that you use regularly, and dialog is the worst but you get into a rhythm with that. It also gives you a pause between each speaker to consider what they might say next, so perhaps it is a blessing in disguise. For the Indian character names I am just using an easy placeholder word that I will go back and fix later."

Different methods of dictation

There are two main methods of dictation:

(1) Voice to text in real time

Use a microphone to dictate straight into a text program, and adjust the words on the screen as you go. You may also be using voice commands to do other tasks e.g. open email program, send messages and more.

(2) Dictate now, transcribe later

Use a recording device to record your words now and later have them transcribed. You can send them to a transcription service like Speechpad.com or you can upload them into Dragon Transcription or another program.

I tried real time speech-to-text and struggled, as watching the words appear on the screen kept my critical voice in the foreground. I wasn't able to speed up as I was always concerned with fixing the errors on-screen.

Now I record directly into my Sony recorder and later on, I upload into Dragon Dictate on my Mac which creates a .txt file. I copy and paste that into Scrivener and lightly edit that file. It's usually pretty exact and this is definitely my preferred process now.

Fantasy author Kevin J. Anderson talked about his dictation process in a podcast interview on The Creative Penn:

> "I'm a storyteller. I know my novel. I have it all outlined, the hundred chapters or so blocked out with, maybe three or four sentences each. I live in Colorado so I'm in the mountains. It's very beautiful scenery and I'll go out walking with my digital recorder and just tell the story in my head.
>
> Now, all writers, they think of a sentence and then they type it. Well, **I think of the sentence, then I speak it. I'm going through far fewer steps than somebody who types it because I can just think it and talk.**
>
> Rather than mentally deconstruct the sentences into words, and then break those words down into letters,

and then type those letters on a keyboard so that it comes up on the screen. That's like seven extra steps to type your stuff.

So, I get to go out walking. I can be on a trail somewhere or a smooth bike path and just be away from the telephone, away from the computer, away from the nagging little Facebook icon that wants me to check my Facebook status and Twitter, or whatever. I'm just synced entirely into the story that I'm writing and I usually walk along the trail until I've dictated one chapter. Then I turn around and I have just enough time to dictate another chapter on the way back home.

I email the audio files to a typist who transcribes. Sometimes, I will transcribe it myself if I'm in a real hurry. But I'd rather spend the hour dictating another couple of chapters so that I can move forward."

Listen to the whole interview at:
www.TheCreativePenn.com/kevin

Romance author Elle Casey also talked about her experience in another interview:

"**Before dictation, I used to be tied to my computer** and tied to my bed because that happens to be the most comfortable place for me to write and it's the quietest place. But then, I'm stuck in a bedroom while everybody else is outside enjoying the beautiful weather in Southern France, walking the dogs, and doing all that fun stuff.

So I bought a little Sony Dictaphone that's about half the size of my cell phone and I took one of my dogs for a walk. It was late in the evening, and dark out. I started walking and I realized that **with the dog keeping part of my attention, I could dictate a chapter without really realizing what was going on.** I didn't focus too hard on it, so I let my mind wander.

Now I can take an hour walk with my dog, and I can write 5000 words, whereas 5000 words took me 3-4 hours before. So I have had 15,000 word days just working a few hours. I could literally write a book in two weeks now, start to finish.

That being said, there's always the other side of the coin. It's very rough because first of all, the dictation software doesn't get it exactly right, so you have to go back and polish but also telling a story is a totally different skill than writing a story which is kind of weird.

But there's something going on when you're staring at the screen and you're watching the words versus not seeing the words and just wandering around the Earth somewhere. I have had to build that skill, and it's taken me two months to be a semi-decent storyteller."

Listen to the whole interview at:
www.TheCreativePenn.com/elle

Technical set-up

Speech-to-text technology is improving incredibly fast and will only continue to improve with the mainstream adoption of in-home devices and assistants.

There are different apps and hardware and software options, so you don't need everything listed below. Get started with one variation based on the process you want to use and change as you improve along the way.

Recording device

Your options will depend on how you want to dictate and your budget.

- Use your smartphone to record memos through an app like Voice Memos, Evernote or any recording app. There is also a smartphone Dragon Dictation app which syncs with the cloud.

- Hand-held MP3 recorder. I have the Sony ICD-PX333

- Record straight into your computer/laptop using software like Dragon

Microphone

- Desktop microphone to use when recording straight into your computer. I use the ATR 2100

- Lavalier microphone/lapel mic for standing/walking which you can plug into your MP3 recorder or smartphone

- I just talk straight into my hand-held MP3 recorder and it works well enough. You could also talk straight into your smartphone.

The quality of your microphone will make a huge difference to the accuracy of your transcription, so if you are having a lot of errors, look at improving/upgrading your microphone first.

Method for transforming speech to text

- Use a transcription service like Speechpad or find a transcriptionist yourself if you prefer the human touch.

- Most authors use Nuance Dragon which has PC and Mac versions and is the most developed speech-to-text software around.

- Use free built-in software on your computer. On a Mac, use Edit -> Start Dictation. On a PC, use Speech Recognition. Most smartphones have a dictation function for taking notes, or you can use Evernote or other apps.

Tips for getting started with dictation

"The biggest advice that I would give for you and for other writers to get started with dictation is don't try to write that way. The best way to start is to do notes or brainstorming. Take your recorder and just go for a walk. It's almost like free association."

Kevin J. Anderson

"Dragon thinks very differently than we do. So we think in words, right? But Dragon thinks in phrases. So think about what you're going to say and then speak it with confidence. This makes the punctuation easier, too."

Monica Leonelle, author of Dictate your Book.

"Embrace dictation as a productivity tool. It's a weapon in your writing arsenal and your workflow. Don't treat it like it's something completely alien.

We're familiar with the keyboard, but that isn't necessarily the best input method anyway. Input methods keep changing. We've had the quill, and then we had the pen and then we had the typewriter and now we have the computer keyboard. In the last few years, we've had touch.

I genuinely believe that the next big input method is voice. In the next 10 years, if you're not embracing voice, you will be behind in the same way as if you don't have a smartphone right now, you're missing out on a lot of technological help."

Scott Baker, author of The Writer's Guide to Training Your Dragon

My current thoughts on dictation

I dictated the first draft of my last novel, *Map of Shadows*, and it was a much faster creation process than my usual first drafts. I had it done in 27 writing days (about five weeks' elapsed time) and some days, I got up to 5000 words an hour by dictation.

Because I usually write in public spaces, I booked a room at a local co-working space for two hours a day and dictated there. I had a rough outline of a couple of sentences per scene that I worked through so I knew approximately what I was writing as I went. If I needed to describe a scene, I found examples on the internet and talked about them as I dictated, which replicated my usual research process.

So the writing was faster but the editing was a lot harder. I wrote one chapter on a long walk along the canal and it was a real mess, just a stream of consciousness with some gems in it. It needed a lot of rewriting to make it coherent. I also found my sentences were more passive than my usual writing, so the edit was a lot harder as I had to rewrite sentences.

Then I got the manuscript back from my editor, Jen, who commented, "It really feels like the shift has reinvigorated writing for you."

So my writing voice has changed through the process of dictation, and perhaps made my story fresher and my 'voice' clearer. I also improved during the course of dictating the manuscript, so the later chapters are cleaner than the earlier ones. It was a new genre, a new world and new characters, so it's likely that the first draft would have been a bit of a mess even if I had typed it, since I am mostly a pantser.

It's also worth noting that the other novel I dictated, *Destroyer of Worlds*, was a finalist for the International Thriller Writer awards Best Ebook Original 2017, so the finished product can certainly be a good read!

I'm intending to continue writing with dictation and aim to make it an integral part of my creative process.

Questions:

- Why do you want to dictate? What are the benefits you're seeking? Write down your reasons because that will carry you through the resistance!

- What's stopping you from dictation? How can you get over those hurdles?

Resources:

- *Dictate your Book* – Monica Leonelle

- *The Writer's Guide to Training your Dragon* – Scott Baker

- *Foolproof Dictation* – Christopher Downing

- Interview with Monica Leonelle on How to Dictate your Book: www.TheCreativePenn.com/monicadictate

- Interview with Scott Baker on How to Use Dictation to Write Faster and Stay Healthy: www.TheCreativePenn.com/scott

2.8 The active writer mindset

"Being active every day makes it easier
to hear that inner voice."

*Haruki Murakami, What I Talk About
When I Talk About Running*

Getting more active is perhaps the single best thing you can do as a sedentary writer. It has been found that only about 1 in 5 people (21%) in the USA get the recommended levels of physical activity.

There is a tremendous amount of pleasure from moving.

It could be a vigorous walk up a hill or a gentle stroll through streets and a park. It might be a yoga session or a game of squash with friends. A round of golf stolen on a summer's evening, a sweaty session in the gym, or a few laps of the pool will all give you a boost. There are an infinite number of ways to get moving, to be physically active and have rich experiences of activity. It was common advice in The Healthy Writer survey. Take breaks, be active, find the activity that suits you and do it regularly.

If you are going to get more active you also need to consider your own reasons for it.

What are your goals?

Do you just want to be able to play football with your kids?

Perhaps you want to be able to walk up a flight of stairs or walk up the local hill without feeling floored by the effort.

Maybe you are still harboring ambitions to run a local race or swim a mile in the pool. You might just want to feel a little more comfortable in your skin or you are shocked at how you looked in a photo.

You will need to understand your own reasons if you are going to get your active mindset right.

Moving more can find its form in all sorts of different activities. There is no right way.

It doesn't have to be running. For many people just setting out to be more active running is likely to be too much, too soon. It is not for everyone in any case. It does get mentioned frequently here because it is the exercise I do most but all the advice is transferrable to your preferred activity.

If you are going to get more active in your daily life, then you need to adopt an active mindset. You need to start looking at the world slightly differently. Those of us living in the so-called developed world need to fight against public spaces that tend to discourage movement and encourage us to spend more of our time in a car. One of the best ways to build movement as a habit is to seek opportunities for it and to appreciate its simple joys.

"The best exercise *for you* is the one you'll actually do. The one you look forward to. The one you *enjoy.*"

Kristine Kathryn Rusch, from KrisWrites.com

It is worth considering your existing relationship with exercise and activity. Identify where you are now on this list below. Be honest. There's no one watching! You have to know where you are and where you want to be, in order to make a change.

Completely inactive

You are not even walking much. Running is unimaginable torture and you have no desire to take it up or it feels like an unobtainable goal.

You know that exercise could help you, but perhaps you don't know where to start or you feel too embarrassed to take it up. You would like to do more to get the benefits but you haven't enjoyed doing physical exercise in the past. So you keep putting it off.

If you fall into this group, then you probably have the most to gain by moving more.

There is no right answer for the type of exercise you should do. One of the first things you could do to is start by keeping a record of your activity. Fitness trackers work well for this, but you shouldn't feel you have to spend money to do something that is, at its heart, free. The next chapter has some more strategies that can help.

Inactive

You are doing far less activity than you would like. You would be open to trying other kinds of more vigorous exercise like running but it still feels a long way off at this point. You would like to build up to it.

You may benefit from setting specific goals but the first aim should be to build and consolidate your habits. The advice in the next chapter will still be important to you but you may be able to move on quicker.

Intermittently active

You have enjoyed doing physical activities and exercise in the past but you have not managed to be very consistent. You may be in a lull at the moment or you are aware that you have not managed to develop good habits around exercise and activity.

This is the group that is most likely to have a gym membership but often be on the brink of canceling. You may hang onto it as your exercise waxes and wanes.

Consolidating your exercise habit should be your number one priority.

Identify factors in your life that have resulted in you falling off the wagon. You need to look at your habits and try to identity ways in which you can be more consistent in your approach.

Active

You don't need much motivation as you have already experienced the benefits of being physically active. If anything you want to ensure you keep grooving in the good habits and want to avoid falling back into old bad habits.

You might need to consider further consolidation and planning for times when your activity dips (for instance when approaching a deadline or over vacation periods when you have extra family commitments).

Also consider whether you are getting enough rest. Be careful not to over-train, as it can be damaging to your health and creativity.

You may benefit from setting a challenge and a goal.

You are already in the minority of people who meet and probably exceed the recommended amounts of activity. Take pride and encourage your friends and fellow writers!

"Most runners run not because they want to live longer, but because they want to live life to the fullest."

*Haruki Murakami, What I Talk About
When I Talk About Running*

Exercise-related challenges and goals

Goals are important to many people but I don't find races and events work brilliantly well for me and it's certainly not necessary to be active.

In recent years I've done just three events: the Snowman Triathlon in the hills of Snowdonia in Wales; the Alpe d'Huez triathlon that cycles up the famous French hairpins to the ski station; and the Ring of Steall SkyRace in Scotland (29km and 2500m of running). They were all hard but were within my limits given the amount of training I do. Just.

I find that I get very stressed by these events. In two out of the three races I had terrible stomach related problems including cramps and nausea. I didn't enjoy them and my gut highlighted how much they stressed me out. I *never* get these issues when I go out by myself and I love exercising in the hills. The events were both firmly in the category of type 2 fun, the variety that you only enjoy in retrospect. So, I'm wary about committing to events now.

Many people will find themselves hugely motivated by their goals. For example, Joanna is a goal-orientated person, as she outlines in Chapter 2.12 about walking a double-ultra-marathon in a weekend. This personality type always need something to get them out, to force them out the door when they don't quite feel like it. It could be a 5K race or a sponsored walk. It doesn't matter. It could be anything.

So, as with the writing life, it's about knowing yourself. If you are in that group, then carefully select goals that are realistic. Don't feel they are necessary to be active and enjoy exercise. It's about your well-being, and you are not compelled to do anything.

Exercise is too painful for me

Developing an active mindset involves recognizing the difference between pain and discomfort.

Many people have very negative associations with exercise. It could be psychological, with memories of humiliation during sport at school. It could be the memory of serious and unpleasant physical pain through exercising. The mantra of "pain is weakness leaving the body" isn't helpful and I don't believe that doing exercise should be painful.

However, I do know that there can be times of significant discomfort.

For me, I know it sometimes hurts a little to run uphill and I know my legs will ache afterwards. I wouldn't call it pain, it's an enjoyable discomfort, but it can be a fine line and recognizing your own limits comes with experience.

Exercising through pain is rarely a good idea. Exercising through a level of discomfort is probably going to be needed at some point.

This leads us into one of the most important aspects of getting fitter.

The most important principle about getting fit

So here it is: *you do not get fitter during the actual exercise.*

Exercising makes you fitter by putting a strain on your system. Your body then reacts to this stress through our incredible adaptive mechanisms. This is the idea of progressive overload. You need to do enough to get your body to recognize it is under additional stress and then the magic is in the recovery.

This highlights an important point about doing exercise to get fitter. You need progressive overload to get fitter and you then *need time and rest* in which to adapt.

It is the adaptation that makes the difference. It is one of the most remarkable qualities of skeletal muscle and all the muscles that move us around that they have this capability to change and adapt. The same is true for our hearts and lungs and their ability to move oxygen around our system to get to the muscles. All of these can, and will, adapt and improve if you put them under some strain.

It's brilliant. It is also forgotten by many people.

If you just go out and run or bike or lift weights over and over again, you never give yourself the chance to adapt before you are broken. You can't get fit in one day.

This is relevant to anyone who is aiming to get a bit fitter. It takes time.

Be patient, persistent, and consistent. Good principles for the writing life in general.

"I've found that maintaining a regular running schedule has helped enormously with controlling my stress levels, while giving my brain plenty of creative brainstorming time to get myself out of plot holes and writing slumps."

Carrie McAllister, The Healthy Writer survey

Questions:

- What are your reasons for wanting to get more active? Write them down.

- What activities have you enjoyed in the past? Could you get back to them again now?

- Do you have negative associations with exercise? What are they? How can you tackle those and be more active?

- Do you have any goals with your exercise? Are they realistic? Have you shared them with anyone else? Will that help you?

Resources:

- NerdFitness.com. A fitness website for nerds and average joes. There are lots of different websites and communities online that will help with fitness and diet, so you are likely to find one that resonates with you and fits with your body and choices. This one made me laugh, so I thought I'd include it here, but it's just a start.

- *What I Talk About When I Talk About Running* – Haruki Murakami

2.9 Strategies for the sofa-bound

> "A long dog walk is the best remedy for
> all my writing issues!"
>
> *Steven Hayward, The Healthy Writer survey*

The UK, USA and Australia all make similar recommendations on the minimum amount of exercise a person should take for good health. All the guidelines are presented in several different ways, so there is a lot of flexibility if you are into different sports such as swimming, or tennis, or cycling.

In the UK the recommendation for adults aged 19-64 is 150 minutes of moderate aerobic activity per week. That might break down into five walks (if that's your thing) of about 30 minutes each in a week. The USA also recommends 150 minutes of physical activity spread throughout the week.

There is some evidence that 'weekend warriors' who do the bulk of their exercise in a binge at the weekend get the same benefits, so it doesn't always have to be split across the week. In addition, the guidelines also recommend strength exercises on two or more days that work the major muscles in the body.

All the guidelines emphasize that *doing more than the minimum will give additional health gains.*

These recommendations do get tweaked from time to time.

Try searching "physical activity guidelines <your country>" and Dr Google will steer you in the right direction. If you are older than 64 or younger than 19 then all the countries have age-specific advice that you should check out.

So, if you fall into the completely inactive category, then aim for 150 minutes, or two and a half hours, of moderate exercise every week. That could be 30 mins x 5 sessions a week.

Start small and build up

If you have been completely inactive then there is no need to rush in with unrealistic goals. And rather than jumping straight to over two hours of exercise, it may be something to work toward incrementally.

Remember that exercise is based on your own ability. You are not expected to walk, run, cycle or swim at a set pace. It is all about raising your own heart rate to a certain level (really quite a modest one). The aim should be to build your activity.

At the start, it may be enough to simply get up and do a few steps every hour. Wearable fitness trackers like a Fitbit will buzz if you don't do any steps for a user-defined period of time.

What is moderate aerobic activity?

A brisk walk fits the bill here. It should be the kind of exercise that makes you feel pretty darn warm, and if not outright sweating you should certainly be glowing. You can do something similar on a bicycle.

Notice how no one is suggesting a speed. This is all about you. You should be able to hold a conversation, and that does suggest you should be able to dictate, so you don't necessarily have to lose writing time.

However, there is also an argument for enjoying the activity itself, being mindful and relaxing into it, rather than furiously multi-tasking. Either works.

> "Whenever I'm feeling off, I step away from my computer and take my dog for a walk. It calms me and energizes my thought process."
>
> *Janine, The Healthy Writer survey*

Measure what activity you are doing

If you take up walking or some other kind of physical exercise, then make a note of what you have been doing. This could be as simple as recording the time you spend walking, cycling, or doing any activity that counts as moderate exercise. There are dozens of apps that will do it for you as well. They can track you using GPS data and give you a breakdown of every detail. If that's your thing then go ahead, but don't let these become a barrier to exercise. Going for a walk doesn't involve any tech beyond a pair of shoes and some layers of clothing, but technology can offer some help to measure your activity levels.

Get a fitness tracker

One of the simplest ways to measure your levels of activity is to get some wearable technology. It used to be that a simple pedometer was the only method for measuring steps, but nowadays there is a smorgasbord of wearable technology that will do the job. You can buy a simple watch fitness tracker for just $30.

You will need a smartphone to connect it and, of course, you can spend a lot more but the cheap ones will often do the job and get you started. It is also possible to use your phone in your pocket as most of them have built-in accelerometers. It's a good way to start but be aware that some research suggests the accuracy of phone-based step counters can leave much to be desired.

Measure your steps

Measuring steps is a brilliantly simple and effective way to start the process of getting yourself more active.

There's good evidence that using a pedometer will increase your physical activity, reduce blood pressure, and help weight loss. A typical number of steps to aim for is around 10,000 a day. It sounds a lot but it can be done in with a modest amount of walking each day.

There is no 'right' number of steps but research has also suggested that having a step goal like this gives better results.

I (Euan) find that it works well for me. If I am out running, then I blast through the steps easily. I'm not worried about those days. It's the days where I am stuck at my desk and I have no plans for a run, cycle or swim that cause a problem. That can be three days a week and I've noticed that I can often get stuck at around a dismal 5000-6000 steps. Getting out for a brief walk at lunchtime is usually enough to raise my steps and I feel much better for it.

There is evidence that pedometers can be an effective method to get people more active and promote weight loss.

One trial gave pedometers to women who were overweight. The women who had the pedometers lost an average of 8.7kg over the three-month study and the control group without pedometers lost just 1.4kg. The women with the pedometers increased their daily average steps by nearly 1000 steps over the course of the study. What gets measured gets managed.

There is also good evidence that pedometers can help people with chronic musculoskeletal disorders and people with type 2 diabetes. They help increase levels of physical activity and a couple of the studies in the diabetes review suggested improvements in blood glucose as well.

"I wear a Fitbit health tracker to remind me to get up and move at least once an hour. It has been very beneficial."

Rhonda, The Healthy Writer survey

2.10 The active writer: Three golden rules

"Yoga saved my back. Walks saved my mental health. Bodywork helps manage my long-standing RSI issues."

Ethan Freckleton, The Healthy Writer survey

If you are serious about getting active, then let me (Euan) offer three golden rules that can be applied to people at all levels. It doesn't matter if you are just setting out to become more active or if you are planning your next marathon. They'll stand you in good stead to build a lifestyle that embraces physical activity.

Golden rule #1: Beware comparisonitis

You are doing this for you.

We all have different hopes and aims from our activity so don't get sucked into comparisons with others. If you suffer easily from comparisonitis then social media sites can be toxic. They can also be a great source of support, a community that helps you get out and keeps you motivated. But remember that the only person you need to worry about is yourself.

I'm prepared to wager that you don't regard yourself as a better person if you finish ahead of someone during a running race or if you walk to the top of a hill quicker than them. Why then would you regard yourself as a failure if you finish behind them? Read Joanna's experience during an ultra-marathon in Chapter 2.12 to help you put it into perspective.

So, beware comparisonitis, but I do think it is reasonable to set modest personal goals.

Most people are aware of the SMART acronym for these: Specific, Measurable, Achievable, Realistic, and Time-bound. Don't just aim to be 'more active' in some vague way. Set a specific goal. Many people will tell you of the benefit of making a commitment to that goal. It could be to your family, or in public, or it could be to your writing group or similar. It's the same principle as finishing a book. Setting word count targets and a publishing deadline can help you make it to achieving your writing goals.

I'm a strong advocate for keeping a record of your activity. It's the single best way to keep yourself accountable and build a habit for the long term. However, if you are the type of person who feels a sorrowful pang when you see someone else's achievements on Facebook, do yourself a favor and stay away from the more social aspects of the various apps. And if you get overtaken while out of a walk, or a run, or cycle, then don't let that phase you. You are out there doing your thing. For you. For your own reasons.

Golden rule #2: Don't get injured

For most people, other than those competing at the highest levels, the most important thing about your exercise is that it is consistent. You can't do that if you are lying on the couch with your calf muscle shredded or your knee joints ground to a paste. You need to build up to it.

Of course, anybody can be unlucky. Stuff does happen.

You can twist an ankle on some uneven ground or break a wrist slipping on ice. You may be carrying old injuries or illnesses that affect the exercise you can do. We have to work around those, but don't be the architect of your own downfall. Don't let a rush of enthusiasm lead you into unsustainable volumes or methods of exercise.

This where you need to listen to your body and try to pick up the signals. Pushing through some discomfort is reasonable. Getting injured through pushing yourself too far is a disaster. It is also ridiculously common.

It's not normal or necessary to get injured being physical active. You need to make exercise a habit over the long term and build up to bigger goals slowly. You can't develop a habit if you are broken.

Golden rule #3: It's not about the bike

Don't get seduced into buying lots of shiny new pieces of gear.

Most physical activity is fundamentally cheap. You need almost nothing to go out walking. Just a pair of shoes that won't strip your feet of flesh and will hopefully keep them warm and dry. Most people have those already.

You need very little specialist kit to go running. I would encourage good footwear. When I first started running back in 1992 I bought a pair of cheap and nasty Hi-Tec Silver Shadows. There were exactly the same trainers that the British Army issued to all recruits. Within a few weeks of running I developed shin splints. The pain down the front of my shins stopped me running for a couple of weeks. I bought a proper pair of running shoes and never had problems again.

Running shoes are the biggest investment but if you're prepared to wear last season's colors then you can usually find a bargain. You will need some shorts or leggings that won't rub your thighs raw. Women need to invest in a decent sports bra. A hat and gloves are useful if it's cold. But they don't need to be specially bought. Wear what you have.

The costs of cycling can quickly mount up, but don't forget the law of diminishing returns. Spending $4000 on a carbon fiber bike rather than $500 on a secondhand bike will not make you eight times faster. It is exactly the same amount of physical effort when going slower on your old bike as it is on one that costs more than a small car. It will make zero difference to your ability to exercise.

Don't let equipment dictate terms to you.

Questions:

- Are you prone to comparisonitis? Are you putting yourself under too much pressure with unrealistic goals that aren't SMART?

- Are you the type of person who likes to feel the burn and push yourself hard? Are you putting yourself at more risk of injury?

- How much money do you spend on equipment for sport? Do you worry that you need a lot of gear to get started? Could it be a form of procrastination?

Resources:

- *Sorted: The Active Woman's Guide to Health* – Juliet McGrattan

- *Your Pace or Mine?: What Running Taught Me About Life, Laughter and Coming Last* – Lisa Jackson

2.11 The running writer: Three rookie errors

"Exerting yourself to the fullest within your individual limits: that's the essence of running, and a metaphor for life — and for me, for writing as whole."

Haruki Murakami, What I Talk About
When I Talk About Running

Running is not for everyone, but many writers have found it to be a wonderful way to stay active and counteract the sedentary nature of the work. I (Euan) love running, so this chapter is for those writers who might want to try it too. Just skip over this if it's not your cup of tea.

If you are new to exercise then here are three basic errors that will make a significant difference to your training. Get these right and you will see major improvements in relatively short periods of time. You will minimize the risk of injury and you might just enjoy it. If you are new to running, then come back to Error #2 later.

Error #1: Going too fast

This is common to almost all runners, even the very experienced, but it is particularly important for newbies. It is possibly the single biggest reason that people hate running and never manage to get into it.

People run too fast and end up bent over, panting for breath, and hating the experience. They are in pain.

But it shouldn't be this way.

A common method of measuring this is to say that you should be able to hold a conversation with somebody.

Try it next time you're out for a run. You'll find that it is much slower than you expected. Do not be demoralized. You may be itching to go faster. Don't. You may be embarrassed to be running as slowly. You may even have to resort to a fast walk. That's OK. Do not go faster.

You are still getting massive cardiovascular benefit at the conversational level. The great advantage of going more slowly and exercising in this heart-rate zone is that you will be nowhere near as tired as you would have been if you try to push it harder. That means that your leg muscles will be less sore and you will feel fresher and recover quicker. Rather than going for a run and feeling completely wrecked for four days afterwards, you'll have some mild discomfort but feel reasonably normal the next day. There may even be a chance that you'll feel positively enthusiastic about going out again.

Running at the right speed feels good!

The only thing that makes people run faster is some expectation that they put on themselves or that gets put on them by people around them. You are not aiming to stride out like double Olympic champion Mo Farah hitting the bell. You may only be able to manage a fast walk because even a gentle jog will make you too breathless. You have to get over that and shut out the world around you.

Remember Golden Rule #1: Beware comparisonitis. Those who go out and thrash themselves for two or three runs can't maintain that habit for the long term.

Error #2: Going too slow

This one is only applicable for more advanced exercisers.

Once you get yourself moving and you've picked up a little bit of an exercise habit, then you may start to think about pushing it further and getting quicker. It is worth mentioning as you may feel you have no chance of improving your running if you continue to exercise in the easiest heart-rate zones.

When it comes to going faster with running what you have to do is run really fast. For short bursts. Yes, welcome to the fantastic world of intervals and repetitions (reps). These are the real gold when it comes to getting fast at running.

The idea is that you take period of time and get yourself fully warmed up. That might be a 15 or 20 minute jog during which you take it easy and you make sure the blood is flowing and you have a bit of a sweat on. Some gentle stretches are a good idea.

Once you are fully warmed up, you are then ready to do some intervals. These can be done just about anywhere and you don't need to have any special facilities. Having said that, if you have a local running track, then you will have a better idea of exactly how far you are running for each interval, but it's certainly not crucial.

For many years I did these around a local football pitch, which was ideal as I was running on soft grass. Nowadays

I tend to do any interval sessions on the hillside and so I incorporate them into my regular fell run.

So, everything is ready … Let the fun begin.

Let's take an interval set of 5×100 m. The aim is that you will run that hundred meters fast. Not an all-out sprint but a sustainably fast pace. You will then have a break where you might jog back along the 100m or you'll just jog for 30 seconds. You then run another hundred meters at the same pace. You keep on doing this until you are finished with the session.

While these seem deceptively straightforward on paper, they do bring in a whole new dimension of discomfort. It will be approximately half-way through your first interval session when you begin to wish you had taken up knitting. The only crumb of comfort you can cling onto during these intervals is that they will give you remarkable results in terms of your overall fitness. You'll be stronger, faster, and mentally hard as nails.

Remember, they are absolutely not to be undertaken until you have a solid base of aerobic fitness. Remember Golden Rule #2: Don't get injured.

Error #3: Taking it too seriously

This is a common error that many runners make. Particularly once you start throwing in a few faster runs and intervals. It all gets so serious and determined.

Running should be tremendous fun.

When you see kids tearing around a playground, screaming and laughing, reveling in physical activity, they aren't thinking about whether or not their heart rates are in zone one or two or whether they are at their anaerobic threshold.

They are not thinking about the training benefits they are getting and the adaptation that is going to occur.

They are not fretting about how they are going to humble brag on Facebook later about the run. They are just simply in the moment, enjoying themselves. They are the ultimate mindfulness machines when it comes to physical exercise. You need to be the same.

We should be aiming for the uninhibited, unselfconscious freedom of enjoying our bodies in the moment. I like running in the hills and it is those experiences that are burned into my mind. Tearing down the side of a hill, legs thumping, arms whirling, with a face-splitting grin. Those are the memories that will never leave me.

So, that means you shouldn't go out and buy an expensive GPS watch, you shouldn't obsess about your status on Strava. You should try to get yourself an exercise habit that means you feel good about yourself and brings you pleasure. It won't be perfect every day but if you feel the joy is lacking and it is just becoming another item on your list, then try the session below.

"The aim of effortless exercise is not to win, not even to compete. Neither is it to get fit, lose weight, or improve body shape, though all of these will happen. There's no score to keep, no technique to master. There's just the body, aware of itself, enjoying movement for its own sake."

Orna Ross, Go Creative series

Just for fun: the Ultimate Recovery Run

Sometimes, you need to run without a watch. Leave it at home.

Most people take a stopwatch and even that is not necessary. Go out and enjoy it.

One thing you can do if you find yourself getting oppressed by the need to record and document and analyze your training is to leave it all behind. Pull on your trainers and leave your phone at home. If you can, avoid even looking at the clock before you leave. You don't want to know anything about your time. And then run something called *fartlek*. It's a Swedish word that means 'speed play.'

The idea is that you don't run a consistent pace, and it's often more fun in a group. You might sprint from one lamppost to the next, then you jog very slowly for the 400m down by the canal, then you'll pick it up for the next 5-10 minutes before settling into a jog. Or, what the heck, just walk for a bit. Then go again as if you've just been tagged in a playground game.

The aim is not to have a fixed pattern: you go slow, you go fast, you just run around and enjoy yourself. Sometimes I do some skipping, sometimes I do some sideways bouncing. Listen to some music if it helps. Dance a bit. It really doesn't matter. The idea is you simply go out and immerse yourself in the activity without worrying about anything else. Just enjoy it.

"It's important to switch off, and running also allows you to access parts of your creative brain that are otherwise hard to get to."

Mark Dawson, The Healthy Writer survey

2.12 Lessons learned about writing from walking 100km

In July 2016, I (Joanna) completed the Race to the Stones, 100km from Lewknor to Avebury standing stones along The Ridgeway, one of Britain's oldest walking trails. I did it over two days, so I walked 50km on Saturday, camped and then walked the final 50km on Sunday, resulting in a double ultra-marathon.

Despite weeping with pain in the final kilometers, I finished it with a (tired) smile on my face. My feet were a mess of burst blisters, my muscles ached, and I was exhausted for a week afterward, but it was well worth the effort.

Since then, I have done 50k along the Cotswold Way in one day and have booked for the Isle of Wight Challenge, 104km around the island in two days, and this time I'll be looking after my feet!

I now walk 10-15km most weekends (for fun!) and do longer training walks, as well as going on multi-day walking holidays, most recently in the Dolomite mountains of northern Italy.

Walking has helped my fitness levels, but it's also critical for my mental health.

I feel the difference when I walk regularly. Focusing on the more basic aspects of life – water, shelter, warmth, food, putting one foot in front of the other – help to put things in perspective. I stop worrying about book sales and comparisonitis when I'm watching a heron fish on the edge of the canal, or listening to the rain on my hood and the click of my poles on the path. I come up with ideas for stories or things I want to share. If I'm with Jonathan, we talk for hours and make decisions about our life together while walking, or I might listen to an audiobook or podcast.

Walking is one of the most important practices in my life, alongside regular writing, and now yoga. Here are some lessons I've learned from walking longer distances that relate to writing.

(1) Deadlines, specific written goals, and accountability help you achieve more

One of the problems with statements/resolutions like "I will exercise more," or "I will write more," is that they are not specific enough and they don't have a deadline.

Booking an event like Race to the Stones, or committing to a specific date for getting your book to an editor, means you are far more likely to achieve that goal. I booked the race when we moved out of London to Bath. I needed to get out in nature and walk more after years of living in a built-up urban area. Having a goal made me walk farther and train harder than just walking for fun.

Being accountable also helps, and I announced the event on my podcast and blog, as well as on social media. When I wanted to give up on the walk at around 77km, I thought about what people would think if I didn't make it. That distance might have been impressive anyway, but in my mind, it was important to be accountable to setting and completing the goal.

So if you're struggling to finish a book, or want to achieve more with your health, set a goal and a deadline and tell people about it.

(2) It's good to have a goal, but training (and the journey) is the point

One of the reasons for moving out of London was to focus on our health, get out into nature more and do more exercise. I set the Race goal so I would have something to train for, and that helped me extend my walks in the months leading up to the event.

I can now happily do 30km in a day, and anything less than 10km feels like a stroll, rather than a walk. You can find me regularly walking the Kennet & Avon Canal path, my favorite walk as there's always something going on and lots of wildlife and birds along the way.

The 100km race was a high point, but it's been the long training walks that have made the most difference to my life. I thought I would dictate more but actually, my mind goes fallow. It seems that I don't even think, especially after about 20km when I start to get tired. It's walking meditation and for someone who is always 'doing,' this mental break has been great for me.

These big walks take up the entire day when I just disconnect and walk, and often the day after, I have a creative burst. After 32km a few weekends ago, I ended up writing ideas for five more fiction books and how they would work together across three different series.

The Race to the Stones was like the publication of a book – a high point in many ways, a low point in others – but the process of walking for training, or the process of creation and writing along the way is the real benefit.

(3) Stamina builds up over time as you practice

You can't get up tomorrow and walk 100km unless you have built up your muscles and stamina over time.

When we moved to Bath, 10km felt like a stretch, and now it's a stroll to a coffee shop on the aqueduct and back. I've been walking several times a week with distances that have grown as time has passed. We also do multi-day walking trips, like in the Alpujarras in southern Spain.

In the same way, you can't sit down and write for hours every day without building up to it. Writing is a surprisingly tiring activity. Your brain uses a lot of energy creating things, and your body will suffer unless you get used to it and introduce some healthy working practices, as we've covered in this book.

It will also feel intimidating to sit down for hours and 'just write.' You have to work up to it. Like walking, start with small distances/times and work up to longer periods as you get used to it.

(4) You need a support team, but no one can do the steps (or the words) for you

Writing is considered a lonely practice … and so is walking. Or at least they can be!

I like solitary walking and also do day walks with Jonathan, but for the Race to the Stones, there was a whole event management team. Plus Jonathan played backup, ferrying me to the event very early and picking up the pieces at the messy end.

I did the steps with my own two feet, but I couldn't have done it without backup support. In the same way, 'self-publishing' is a misnomer because we all need a team. I work with a number of professionals in my creative business and value them highly. We all need professional editors and cover designers at the very least!

(5) There are fun parts ... but some of it will be hell!

There were beautiful moments on The Ridgeway – cresting a hill to see a field of wildflowers stretching into the distance, or the expanse of sky and soaring birds overhead. But the human body is not happy doing 100km in a weekend and it hurt a lot.

Just like writing.

Sometimes it's fun and ideas explode, and words stream onto the page. And sometimes it's like walking that last 30km. Every step and every word is difficult.

(6) Don't compare yourself to others. The Race is only ever with yourself.

2000 people started the Race to the Stones. The fastest time was just over 8 hours, running straight through.

I came in at 25 hours 38 mins, arriving in the last batch of people at 8.10pm on Sunday. I walked nearly 12 hours on Saturday and 14 hours on Sunday. The longest time anyone took was 33 hours 32 mins.

But many people didn't *finish* the whole 100km, so although I was 'slow,' I still came in ahead of them.

The point is that I was never racing the super-fit ultra-marathoner at the front of the pack. And I am not 'better' than the people who did 50k or didn't finish because it hurt too much. I just wanted to make the finish – which I did.

You can't go at the pace of the seasoned ultra-marathoner on your first event. Just like you can't expect to achieve great things with your first book and compare yourself to someone like Stephen King who has been writing for 50+ years.

Quit comparing yourself to others and go at your own pace. Run/walk – or write – your own race.

(7) Follow the path others have set before you

The Ridgeway is one of England's oldest walking paths, and every step I took had been taken by many more before me, both on the race day and for several thousand years before.

I would have been stupid to try and forge my own path through the undergrowth and forests and fields of wheat. I needed to follow the path others had set and the clear course markers along the way.

In the same way, you don't have to write and publish and

market your book on your own. You don't have to hack away the undergrowth. There are many of us who share our journeys so you can follow and (hopefully) have an easier time of it.

(8) It's worth spending some money to get the right gear for specific events

At the start of the Race to the Stones, I saw some people in basic trainers and gym clothes with little bottles of water. Other people wore brand new shoes that hadn't been worn in. Most of those people dropped out pretty soon.

I certainly made some mistakes, but I had been training in my gear and some of the most important included:

- **Multiple pairs of socks**. I like thousand mile socks, which have two layers, or I wear two pairs – a thin pair and then a thicker pair on top. My top tip is to change socks at every rest stop and deal with any sore points early on. I now take 4-5 pairs per day and change them every 10km on the longer walks.

- **Walking shoes** (heavy boots weren't needed for this type of terrain). Mine are Merrell and I'd been walking in them for months so they were well worn in.

- **Walking poles**. Mine are Trekmates Peak Walker but Leki are also a popular brand. Walking with poles protects your knees and with the bumpy path at points, I was glad to have them to stop my (very) wobbly moments. Poles have been shown to reduce fatigue and improve endurance, and they also prevent 'sausage fingers,' which happens if your hands swing by your sides for hours on end.

- **Blister plasters**. Treat sore patches *before* they become blisters and also invest in foot pads for the later kilometers as well as thicker tape that you can just leave on.

- **Stronger painkillers**. When I was weeping with pain at 66km, I took some, and they got me to the finish. Obviously these are not for long-term use but if you want to get through short-term pain, it might be worth it.

In the same way, I recommend authors spend money on professional editing regardless of how they want to publish, and if self-publishing, invest in professional cover design. Yes, it can be free to write and publish a book, but investing in these two things will make your experience (and the reader's) much better!

9) A lot of people give up along the way. Persistence is the key to success.

I didn't even realize that you *could* give up until around 77km!

Many people were injured out or chose only to do 50k (which is still an ultra-marathon!), or just decided the pain wasn't worth it. I phoned Jonathan at one of the rest stops and even though I was crying with pain, he said that if I gave up at that point, I would only need to do it again another year, so I might as well finish. Tough love, but I needed it.

This attrition rate is the same with writing … and blogging, podcasting, and most other things in life.

When I started writing seriously back in 2006, I made early friends online. Most of them have disappeared, with only a few staying the course, and many authors only write one or two books and then give up.

I only have a multi-six-figure business as an author-entrepreneur right now because I have been consistently creating, learning and taking action for years.

Persistence is the secret of success in writing as much as general fitness or finishing ultra-marathons.

So there you go. Walking has a lot of lessons that can apply to writing and the actual practice of walking can help your mental health as well as physical fitness. So what are you waiting for?

2.13 Find a community

"Writing, at its best, is a lonely life … For he does his work alone and if he is a good enough writer he must face eternity, or the lack of it, each day."

Ernest Hemingway

When I started writing seriously back in 2006, I didn't have any friends who were authors. I thought writers were some rare creature, existing on another plain of reality, somewhere I would never be able to reach. I didn't know how to meet other wannabe writers, let alone 'real' authors.

I wasn't lonely, because I'm an introvert and I love being alone. Time on our own is a necessary part of the writer's life. But I was missing a community, other people to learn from and discuss the journey. And I needed new friends, because my corporate life was so different to the creative existence I was trying to cultivate. We all need someone to talk to sometimes.

Here's how I went from billy-no-mates to an active and warm community of author friends.

(1) Join a community online

You are more likely to find a like-minded creative soul online than you are in the next street or even in your town. Let's face it, writers are weird! We all have our crazy obsessions and strange thoughts and we need people who understand what it's like to tune in to this inner life.

I joined Twitter in 2009 and it quickly became a portal to a creative life. This is why it remains my primary social media channel and you can find me there most days @ thecreativepenn. I discovered writers and authors and introvert creatives just like me. I found bloggers and podcasters and people to interview on my podcast, people who helped me realize that there were others like me out there. I was not alone.

In 2012, I became a member of the Alliance of Independent Authors and met a real-life community of writers and independent authors. I liked the ethos of taking control of my writing career and found my home amongst creative entrepreneurs. There's also a Facebook group where new writers ask questions, so wherever you are on the author journey, it's a place you will be welcome.

There are lots more Facebook groups and online communities these days, so whatever genre you write in, there will be one for you. Just make sure the group adds to your creative life, rather than pulling you down. Stay mindful of the reason you're involved and leave if things go toxic.

(2) Find a community locally

If you live in a reasonably large city, there might be a writers' group that will suit you. As above, make sure the group adds to your creative life, as some groups focus on criticism rather than support. Try some out or start your own through a site like MeetUp.com.

"You can't stay in your corner of the Forest
waiting for others to come to you. You have to
go to them sometimes."

A.A.Milne, Winnie-the-Pooh

(3) Go to conventions, conferences or festivals

There are lots of events for writers and creatives. The trick is to go to the SAME events for multiple years running, because then you start to cultivate friendships with people who care about the same things you do.

I've been to Thrillerfest in New York four times now, and there are people I catch up with every year. I also attend CrimeFest in Bristol and London Book Fair every year, and being a regular means I can catch up with friends there.

Yes, it is a financial investment to go to some of these events, but choose carefully, do your research, and make the most of it. Push yourself outside of your comfort zone and talk to people. Try asking, "What do you write?" It's a consistently good conversation starter!

I've found that meeting people in real life changes relationships and is the basis of true friendship over time, which is why I continue to attend conventions annually, even though they are a challenge for my introvert energy management.

(4) Start 'friend' dating

If you meet people online or through writer events, the next step is to suggest a coffee or a wine sometime so you can get to know each other a little better. I call this 'friend dating,' and I've been through it multiple times as I've lived all over the world and cultivated new friendships every time. It's the same if you start a new job, or if you want to find a life partner.

My best friends in real life these days are people I initially met online and then invited for a coffee. Most of those 'friend dates' went nowhere, or became short-term acquaintances on the rollercoaster creative journey, but others are dear friends for life. I also met my husband, Jonathan, online so I can definitely vouch for the process!

One important factor is to only do this with people you feel that you are equal with in some way in terms of your writing life.

So if you haven't finished your first book yet, you are unlikely to be in the same place as someone with twenty books. If you haven't even got a website, you won't be in the same position as someone who has had a site for five years and makes a living online. Your concerns and thoughts will be different and so you're unlikely to find common ground.

Start with writers who are in the same place as you, and over time, you will move along the journey and they will, too, or you will both find new friends.

(5) Combat isolation by getting out of the house. Go somewhere else to write

I worked in open-plan offices and low-rise cubicles for 13 years in my old corporate job. When I finally left, I thought it would be bliss to be alone at home in silence for days on end.

But actually, I found the sudden lack of people and even the routine of the commute very difficult. It was so hard that I ended up joining a library and commuting each day into the city, buying a coffee on the way in as I used to do in the day job and working regular hours in the company of others. I didn't talk to anyone while working – it was a library! – but I did meet other writers for lunch, as per the friend dating approach above.

Six years on, I write most week-day mornings in a quiet café wearing my noise-canceling headphones. I don't talk to people, but the movement and bustle and coffee machine sounds make me feel like I am part of the real world and not entirely existing in my own head.

I highly recommend writing outside of the house, especially if you feel isolated.

Libraries are free and the price of a coffee per hour is cheap office space and good for your mental health. There is a world out there! In fact, a general tip is to make sure you leave the house every day. Get dressed, put outdoor clothes on and walk in the fresh air. Notice the world around you, even if you are silent within it.

(6) Put your writing out in public and attract like-minded people

Everyone judges everyone else.

It's an integral part of life. We have to, because how else can we filter out the people we want to pay attention to, or understand who we might be able to connect with? When people email me or come and talk to me at conferences, I am usually wary until I have checked their online profile and platform. Is there evidence that they are indeed a writer?

This might sound harsh, but I've been blogging since 2008 and a full-time writer since 2011. I know this writing life is hard work. If someone is not committed enough to put their words into the world, either on a blog, in a book, or even on social media, then I'll answer their questions and try to help them, but it's unlikely we will be friends.

If you want to be friends with other writers, you need to write and put your words out there for others to read. Show a piece of yourself, reveal your heart and your life in whatever way suits you. Only in that way will you attract those who feel the same.

> "There are no strangers here;
> Only friends you haven't met yet."
>
> *W.B. Yeats*

2.14 Build well-being with mindfulness

"I learned Vedic meditation to help with many of the issues listed and it has been wonderful. Amongst other things, meditation enables me to let things go rather than brooding on them (e.g. bad reviews, anxiety, etc). It has also helped with my headaches, which were as a result of tension in my neck from sitting at a screen. Finally, it has improved my ability to concentrate so that I can achieve much more in a shorter period of time."

Imogen Clark, The Healthy Writer survey

What is mindfulness?

Jon Kabat-Zinn has offered this definition: "mindfulness is a moment to moment awareness that is cultivated by purposefully paying attention to the present experience, with a non-judgmental attitude."

For something that promises so much it is devastatingly simple.

We just need to live in the moment.

Like any discussion around habits, it quickly becomes clear that most of us go through life with the autopilot taking care of all the navigation. Mindfulness, paying attention, is often sorely lacking. One of the key aspects of mindfulness is that it can change your relationship with negative thoughts. All the emotional reactivity that goes with those thoughts is reduced and you can do some 'cognitive appraisal.' That can then change your perception of events, hopefully in a more positive way.

A million ways to be mindful

I should highlight that mindfulness does not necessarily mean meditation. There are varieties of mindfulness that encompass meditation, but it is not a requirement.

Mindfulness meditation itself originates from Buddhist practices. This origin in a religion may be uncomfortable for some people, but you would be hard-pressed to spot them when it comes to the daily practice of being mindful. Some activities like yoga and tai chi also include mindfulness and meditation into their practice.

There is no right way to be mindful: it is a personal process.

It is also possible to bring mindfulness into your daily life without any significant changes to your lifestyle. Many mindfulness exercises come back to breathing, and it's a very efficient way to draw in your attention and focus.

You can be mindful anywhere.

It could be while sitting in traffic and rather than stressing out about a situation you can't control, you just take a few breaths. It might be while standing outside waiting for a bus, or on a short walk to collect the kids from school.

Some mindfulness exercises will encourage you to be more aware of the world around you. The feeling of warmth on your skin from the sun or the wind ruffling your hair. Other exercises encourage you to be aware of your own body, perhaps the tension across your neck and shoulders, or the pressure where you are clamping your jaw and grinding your teeth. Usually there is one simple aspect to concentrate on.

It is generally about living in the moment more. It encourages you not to wish your life away, appreciate the things that are in front of you now and limit your view for a few moments.

The neuroscience of mindfulness

There is plenty of emerging evidence on what goes on inside that 3lb of brain locked up inside its bony crate when we indulge in a little mindfulness.

In 2010, Yi-Yuan Tang and his colleagues published a paper in the *Proceedings of the National Academy of Science*. It is just three pages long but it was significant. It was the first paper to show that even brief meditation practices could change the structure of the brain.

They found that it took at least six hours, but no more than 11 hours, of practice to start to see changes in a part of the brain known as the anterior cingulate cortex. This helps regulate your emotions and behaviors as well as manage cravings. Mindfulness can change how your brain works in just a few hours.

There is good evidence for the usefulness of mindfulness in a whole array of conditions. These include fatigue, chronic pain, heart disease, type 2 diabetes and insomnia. And there is also evidence that mindfulness can be effective for chronic low back pain.

Mindfulness is proving to be a remarkable tonic for modern life and its stresses. If they could, the public health people would be putting mindfulness in the water.

Is mindfulness just the latest fad?

There is good evidence for the effectiveness of mindfulness. It is not simply a flaky, New Age, on-trend, whack-jobbery intervention for the terminally gullible.

As the evidence has emerged, it has entered the mainstream and is treated quite seriously by healthcare professionals. We are likely to see a lot more mindfulness-based interventions as they make their way into daily medical practice. And, there seems little reason to wait for your healthcare professional to tell you to be more mindful. It is a process you can start straight away.

You can start right now. Try this simple breathing exercise.

Learning to breathe

There are lots of variations on these types of exercises. This is just one example of a simple breathing exercise.

It is not specifically a 'mindful' thing, but it can be used as part of that. It can be particularly helpful for people who are anxious, and exercises like these can be used to manage panic-related symptoms. It only needs to be done for two or three minutes but a daily practice can be very effective.

- Breathe slowly in through the nose and out through the mouth. Try to establish a steady rhythm. It can help to count as you breathe in for 'one, two' then relax as you breathe out for 'one, two, three, four.'

- Place a hand on your tummy just below the ribs. When you breathe in, you should feel your tummy *rise*. This is because your diaphragm, the muscle sitting under your lungs, should be pushing down as your lungs expand.

- As you breathe out your tummy should fall again.

- If you are tense or anxious your breathing might be shallow, and at first your abdomen won't move or it will go in the opposite direction. You might be using the muscles in your upper chest to breathe.

- Concentrate on breaths in for a count of two and slow breaths out for a count of four. (The exact numbers don't matter and some breathing exercises will make inspiration and expiration match.)

- Relax those muscles across the chest and shoulders.

And that's it. It is a remarkably effective and simple exercise. It can also be very useful to do before any kind of public speaking, to try to settle that anxiety and tension you can feel beforehand.

Questions:

- How do you feel about mindfulness? Is it something you would like to incorporate into your routine?

- Do you feel like life is flashing by in a rush? Could you benefit from some moments of calm and mindfulness?

- How could you make mindfulness fit into your daily life? As a minute or two between writing sessions? Or as part of a session such as yoga?

- Do you ever feel tense and anxious or struggle with your breathing? Have you tried some simple breathing exercises?

Resources:

- *Mindfulness for Busy People* – Dr Michael Sinclair and Josie Seydel

2.15 Develop healthy habits for the long term

"My pain was part of my identity, and I was afraid that if I was healthy I would lose my ability to write – I bought into the idea that writers have to suffer. I really wish I could go back and shake some sense into past me. Being healthy has only improved my writing."

Louise Waghorn, The Healthy Writer survey

It is difficult to underestimate the importance of habit when it comes to a healthy lifestyle.

Part 2 of this book is all about developing healthy habits and rebuilding those parts of our lives that are holding us back from being healthy writers.

The evidence shows that much of our lives is spent doing the same thing over and over again. And there are significant advantages to that.

If we had to make individual decisions and weigh up the benefits and risks of every little thing we do, we would be exhausted by the time we got to our breakfast. As it is, most of us roll out of bed and the automatic pilot kicks in so we do exactly the same as we normally do.

There is a lot to be said for having a ritual around your writing.

Some people may make a coffee, they will sit down at a certain time, they will put on a certain piece of music, or perform some other superstitious rite. We all know this is good at putting us into the correct mindset to write and improves our productivity.

However, it is important to recognize that habits will quickly become a problem if they are preventing us from adopting more healthy behaviors. The necessity of breaking bad habits is sometimes as important as the reinforcement and establishment of good habits.

> "Try not to view exercise or sleep as time 'away' from the all-important manuscript but rather as a good investment in the overall creative process!"
>
> *Anon, The Healthy Writer survey*

The problem with habits is that we do them without thinking. That is almost entirely the point of them. Your brain slips into gear, flips control over to the basal ganglia and valuable processing resources are spared for thinking about other things.

An exercise habit

I think of myself as an active person. Naturally so? I'm not so sure.

We all have the same basic physiology, and I'm not sure that people can be *naturally* more inclined. We are all designed for physical exercise in some shape or form. I was active as a child (like most) and played a range of sports but it did drop away in my early adulthood. I had to re-learn the joy of exercise and movement.

Unfortunately it took me another 20 years to turn it into a habit. And while running has always been good for me, the benefits in the past four or five years of entrenching exercise as a habit have far surpassed anything I have experienced before.

If I can do it, then it is achievable for anyone.

It is worth emphasizing that it doesn't involve doing something every single day. I don't exercise every day, my schedule simply isn't flexible enough to accommodate that. And, in all honesty, my body would not cope with it very well either.

I have managed to build good habits, and understanding those has helped nurture the good ones and break down the bad ones.

Understanding habits

There are three core features of habits:

1. Cue or trigger

2. Routine

3. Reward

All of our habits can be broken down into these.

The *cue* is the signal or feeling that triggers the loop.

The *routine* is the action you will take in response to the cue.

The *reward* is the consequence which is often the good feeling.

Email is a classic example. You get a pop up (cue) and open your email app (routine). The reward is that little glow you get when you receive a particularly cool email.

You don't have to get the reward every time, just enough to reinforce the behavior. In fact, if there is a certain random element to the reward and you don't always receive it, that can be particularly powerful in entrenching the habit.

How to develop good habits

Understanding the habit loop can help build good habits as well as break bad ones.

For example, I (Euan) wanted to get out running more regularly during the week. Normally, I get up first so I put my clothes out the night before to avoid disturbing everyone as I clatter around the house.

Cue: I would put out my running kit so I would have to get dressed in it.

Routine: I would then put on my kit without thinking while I was still half-asleep. Once I had the kit on I was already half-way past the procrastination stage. The decision had been taken and I would be much more likely to go for a run.

Reward: Endorphin rush and a good feeling from that morning run.

By simply giving myself a different, unavoidable cue, I vastly increased my chances of going out for a run.

The minimum viable approach to habits

This approach has been advocated by Stephen Guise in his book *Mini Habits*. He presents a compelling case for abandoning goals and concentrating on the development of habits.

A certain amount of willpower is needed to adopt a new behavior. We only have a limited reserve of willpower. Setting the goal target absurdly low makes it tremendously easy to reach. And, most importantly, it is especially useful at overcoming the procrastination associated with difficult tasks. We've all had this experience.

If you set out to write 50 words, you will have far less reluctance to get going than if you know you have to write 1000 words. And, of course, what generally happens is that once you get started, you keep going. The same principle can be applied to almost anything.

Want to establish a core strengthening routine? Set yourself a target of doing a five-second plank.

Want to develop upper body strength? Set yourself the target of doing a single press up.

Want to try to develop a running habit? Set yourself the goal of simply putting on your running kit.

Now, as absolutely ludicrous as that sounds, it will almost certainly result in you doing more exercise on a regular basis, and that leads to a regular routine of the right kind of behaviors.

This approach fits with the habit loop. You might be starting small but you are setting up a process where you are building loops and routines in response to cues that give you rewards.

Habit tracking

There are numerous ways to do track your habits. There are habit tracking apps for phones and computers, but I use a journal as I find it inherently satisfying to color in another little box or put a cross next to the day. It also has the advantage for me that it takes me away from screens for a while and the relentless blue light-bathed existence to which we are all now in thrall.

Breaking bad habits

This is the opposite side to building good habits and is more tricky. At first glance, the reward system doesn't work. The 'don't break the chain' approach to developing good habits appears to, well, break.

The simplest hack for this is to turn around your bad habits and re-frame them as good habits. One of my bad habits was eating in the car. I had to re-imagine this as a positive. Any time I went on my drive home and didn't eat anything, it was recorded as a victory. It was a tick in the box.

I also noticed that I got a secondary reward I wasn't expecting. When I didn't eat car snacks, I took far more pleasure in my evening meal. My enjoyment was significantly heightened because my appetite hadn't been blunted by sugary or fatty snacks.

Building habits when life happens

That's the problem with life. It keeps throwing stuff at us. How do you cope with disruptions to your routine? It could be a work crisis, illness, or just family life.

Travel can throw a spanner in the works. If you are traveling for pleasure and vacation, then you may be less bothered about changes. Conferences and conventions can also cause problems. They can be particularly challenging for introverts, and long-distance travel may leave you fatigued and jet-lagged.

Conserving your energy can be an important element of thriving at these events, particularly if they are multi-day. Give yourself some space. Try to factor in some exercise as well. A decent walk or run can be a brilliant way to take in a new city and recharge your batteries.

Kids are a constant source of disruption. They wake you up in the night and wreck your sleep, they get sick, they need help with homework … Whatever their age, they will find original ways to unsettle your routines.

Your mental approach to all these disruptions is important. Don't let negative thoughts about days where it doesn't quite go to plan affect what you do later in the day, tomorrow, or next week.

The 'don't break the chain' approach to habit-building is very seductive, but it can lead to stress if external factors try to smash it. When life is going through a bobbly patch give yourself a break. Play the long game.

Questions:

- What health-related habits of yours can you identify? Are they good ones or destructive? Can you see triggers and routines in your habits? Can they be tweaked?

- How are your recording your habits?

- How hard are you on yourself if you miss a few days of one of your good habits? Is that having a negative effect on you?

Resources:

- *Mini Habits* – Stephen Guise

- *The Power of Habit: Why we do What we do in Life and Business* – Charles Duhigg

- There are many habit apps: HabitBull, Strides, and Streaks are just three that will track habits for you on iOS and Android devices.

Conclusion:
Your turn. Choose life.

"Be careful about reading health books.
Some fine day you'll die of a misprint."

Markus Herz

Let's face it, you already knew a lot of this stuff.

It's a bit like people who say, "I want to be a writer. What's the secret?"

You know as well as I do that the 'secret' to being a writer is getting your butt in a chair and actually writing (or walking while dictating!).

The secret is the same when it comes to physical health – a good diet, sleep, movement, breathing and regular exercise, getting outdoors in the fresh air, monitoring your moods and being kind to yourself, listening to your body, resting, being mindful, and spending time with friends.

But as with being a writer, you actually have to *choose* to make the changes to your routine in order to fix the problems in your life. Then you have to be persistent and repeat those practices every day.

I (Joanna) can only write this book now because over the last five years, I've made incremental changes that have positively impacted my physical health and I am (mostly) pain-free and a happy writer. Of course, these practices need to be sustained, because physical health is a practice, like writing, that we need to keep focusing on.

A little every day makes a huge difference over the long term, both for writing and for our health.

Here are some options for your next steps.

(1) Make a decision to reduce your immediate pain

It is not acceptable to feel like this and there are ways you can deal with it, but you have to take control and be ready to make some changes.

(2) Write down what hurts and the physical and mental health issues you have right now

Be honest with yourself.

Write down all the niggles which over time may become more significant. What do you want to change about your physical health?

(3) Go through the book again and find some specific suggestions that might help

Write down specific action steps that you will take and put a deadline on them.

(4) Schedule time when you can focus on fixing the health issues that plague you

This might be booking a doctor's appointment, or finding a yoga class, or just putting time for a walk in your calendar so you actually do it instead of putting it off.

(5) Commit to a new practice and then give it time

Don't expect instant results.

Physical health is cumulative, but if you keep persisting you will wake up one day and realize that you've fixed the thing that plagued you – or you have found ways that help you live with it.

(6) Check in with yourself over time

Put a reminder in your calendar so you can revisit the decisions you made and how you might have fallen back into old ways. Health, like writing and creativity, starts to deteriorate if you don't practice regularly.

(7) Balance self-care with kicking yourself into gear

Some days you just need to let yourself rest, to reward yourself for a job well done, to let "the soft animal of your body love what it loves," as Mary Oliver says in her lovely poem, *Wild Geese*.

But other days, you need to drag yourself outside in the cold and get walking, or say no to that slice of yummy cake, or spend time stretching, or learn dictation, or implement any one of the other ideas in this book that will move you toward becoming a healthy writer. It's tough to achieve, but this is part of the journey.

Finally, remember that your body is the only one you have.

It is precious and wonderful, and the home for your remarkable brain that creates words on a page to entertain, educate or inspire others.

You deserve health and happiness, so from both of us, we hope you choose life and wellness on your writer's journey.

Thank you.
Need more help?

Thanks so much for joining us for *The Healthy Writer*. We hope you've found some useful ideas and next steps for your writer's journey.

If you've enjoyed the book, we'd really appreciate a review wherever you bought it to help other writers discover it too.

If you need more help with specific issues, please do see a health professional near you.

If you have suggestions or comments for further editions, please use this feedback form:

www.TheCreativePenn.com/healthyfeedback

Both authors are available for media opportunities or podcast interviews, so please get in touch if you think we can help your audience.

Dr Euan Lawson: euan@euanlawson.com

Joanna Penn: joanna@TheCreativePenn.com

Appendix 1: Bibliography

Sane New World – Ruby Wax

The Artist's Way – Julia Cameron

F-R-E-E Writing with Orna Ross – Orna Ross

Deskbound: Standing up to a Sitting World – Kelly Starret

Ink in the Blood: A Hospital Diary – Hilary Mantel

The Case Against Sugar – Gary Taubes

Bird by Bird – Anne Lamott

On Writing – Stephen King

Gut: The Inside Story of our Body's Most Underrated Organ – Giulia Enders

The Complete Low FODMAP Diet – Dr Sue Shepherd and Dr Peter Gibson

Stealing Fire – Steven Kotler and Jamie Wheal

Drugs - Without the Hot Air – David Nutt

Why We Sleep: The New Science of Sleep and Dreams – Matthew Walker

In Defense of Food: An Eater's Manifesto – Michael Pollan

The Pioppi Diet: A 21-Day Lifestyle Plan – Aseem Malhotra and Donal O'Neill

The Back Sufferer's Bible – Sarah Key

Dictate your Book – Monica Leonelle

The Writer's Guide to Training your Dragon – Scott Baker

Foolproof Dictation – Christopher Downing

What I Talk About When I Talk About Running
– Haruki Murakami

Sorted: The Active Woman's Guide to Health
– Juliet McGrattan

*Your Pace or Mine?: What Running Taught Me About Life,
Laughter and Coming Last* – Lisa Jackson

Mindfulness for Busy People – Dr Michael Sinclair and
Josie Seydel

The Power of Habit – Charles Duhigg

Mini Habits – Stephen Guise

Appendix 2: Selected academic studies

Here are the main studies mentioned in the book by chapter.

7 reasons why writing is great for your health

Emmons RA, and McCullough ME. Counting blessings versus burdens: an experimental investigation of gratitude and subjective well-being in daily life. *J Pers Soc Psychol.* United States; 2003;84(2):377-89

Wood AM, Joseph S, Lloyd J, Atkins S. Gratitude influences sleep through the mechanism of pre-sleep cognitions. *J Psychosom Res* 2009, Jan;66(1):43-8

Kini P, Wong J, McInnis S, Gabana N, and Brown JW. The effects of gratitude expression on neural activity. *Neuroimage.* 2016;128:1-10

1.2 Back, neck and shoulder pain

Chen SM, Liu MF, Cook J, Bass S, Lo SK. Sedentary lifestyle as a risk factor for low back pain: A systematic review. *Int Arch Occup Environ Health* 2009, Jul;82(7):797-806

del Pozo-Cruz B, Gusi N, Adsuar JC, del Pozo-Cruz J, Parraca JA, Hernandez-Mocholí M. Musculoskeletal fitness and health-related quality of life characteristics among sedentary office workers affected by sub-acute, non-specific low back pain: A cross-sectional study. *Physiotherapy* 2013, Sep;99(3):194-200

Sihawong R, Sitthipornvorakul E, Paksaichol A, Janwantanakul P. Predictors for chronic neck and low back pain in office workers: A 1-year prospective cohort study. *J Occup Health* 2016;58(1):16-24

Steffens D, Maher CG, Pereira LS, Stevens ML, Oliveira VC, Chapple M, et al. Prevention of low back pain: A systematic review and meta-analysis. *JAMA Intern Med* 2016, Feb;176(2):199-208

O'Sullivan K, O'Keeffe M, O'Sullivan L, O'Sullivan P, Dankaerts W. The effect of dynamic sitting on the prevention and management of low back pain and low back discomfort: A systematic review. *Ergonomics* 2012;55(8):898-908

1.4 Repetitive Strain Injury (RSI)

van Tulder M, Malmivaara A, Koes B. Repetitive strain injury. *Lancet* 2007, May 26;369(9575):1815-22

Brooks P. Repetitive strain injury. *BMJ* 1993, Nov 20;307(6915):1298

Jacobs K, Foley G, Punnett L, Hall V, Gore R, Brownson E, et al. University students' notebook computer use: Lessons learned using e-diaries to report musculoskeletal discomfort. *Ergonomics* 2011, Feb;54(2):206-19

1.5 Writing with chronic pain

Ballantyne JC, Kalso E, Stannard C. WHO analgesic ladder: a good concept gone astray. *BMJ* 2016:i20–2

Centers for Disease Control and Prevention. Further information on opioid-related deaths in the USA. https://www.cdc.gov/drugoverdose/data/overdose.html

Williams AC de C, Eccleston C, Morley S. Psychological therapies for the management of chronic pain (excluding headache) in adults. *Cochrane Database of Systematic Reviews* 2012, Issue 11. Art. No.: CD007407

Geneen LJ, Moore RA, Clarke C, Martin D, Colvin LA, Smith BH. Physical activity and exercise for chronic pain in adults: An overview of cochrane reviews. *Cochrane Database Syst Rev* 2017;4:CD011279

1.6 Sedentary life and inactivity

Diaz KM, Howard VJ, Hutto B, Colabianchi N, Vena JE, Safford MM, et al. Patterns of sedentary behavior and mortality in U.S. Middle-Aged and older adults: A national cohort study. *Ann Intern Med* 2017, Sep 12

Lear SA, Hu W, Rangarajan S, Gasevic D, Leong D, Iqbal R, et al. The effect of physical activity on mortality and cardiovascular disease in 130,000 people from 17 high-income, middle-income, and low-income countries: The PURE study. *Lancet* 2017, Sep 21

Hagger-Johnson G, Gow AJ, Burley V, Greenwood D, Cade JE. Sitting time, fidgeting, and all-cause mortality in the UK women's cohort study. *Am J Prev Med* 2016, Feb;50(2):154-60

Pulsford RM, Stamatakis E, Britton AR, Brunner EJ, Hillsdon M. Associations of sitting behaviours with all-cause mortality over a 16-year follow-up: The Whitehall II study. *Int J Epidemiol* 2015, Dec;44(6):1909-16

Biddle SJ, Bennie JA, Bauman AE, Chau JY, Dunstan D, Owen N, et al. Too much sitting and all-cause mortality: Is there a causal link? *BMC Public Health* 2016, Jul 26;16:635

Baddeley B, Sornalingam S, Cooper M. Sitting is the new smoking: Where do we stand? *Br J Gen Pract* 2016, May;66(646):258

1.7 Sleep problems and insomnia

Winkelman JW. Clinical practice. Insomnia disorder. *N Engl J Med* 2015, Oct 8;373(15):1437-44

Buysse DJ. Insomnia. *JAMA* 2013, Feb 20;309(7):706-16

Bermudez EB, Klerman EB, Czeisler CA, Cohen DA, Wyatt JK, Phillips AJ. Prediction of vigilant attention and cognitive performance using self-reported alertness, circadian phase, hours since awakening, and accumulated sleep loss. *PLOS One* 2016;11(3):e0151770

Palagini L, Bruno RM, Gemignani A, Baglioni C, Ghiadoni L, Riemann D. Sleep loss and hypertension: A systematic review. *Curr Pharm Des* 2013;19(13):2409-19

Vyas MV, Garg AX, Iansavichus AV, Costella J, Donner A, Laugsand LE, et al. Shift work and vascular events: Systematic review and meta-analysis. *BMJ* 2012, Jul 26;345:e4800

Philip P, Sagaspe P, Moore N, Taillard J, Charles A, Guil-leminault C, Bioulac B. Fatigue, sleep restriction and driving performance. *Accid Anal Prev* 2005, May;37(3):473-8

Lin X, Chen W, Wei F, Ying M, Wei W, Xie X. Night-shift work increases morbidity of breast cancer and all-cause mortality: A meta-analysis of 16 prospective cohort studies. *Sleep Med* 2015, Nov;16(11):1381-7

Killgore WD. Effects of sleep deprivation on cognition. *Prog Brain Res* 2010;185:105-29

1.8 Eye strain, headaches and migraine

Bergqvist UO, Knave BG. Eye discomfort and work with visual display terminals. *Scand J Work Environ Health* 1994, Feb;20(1):27-33

Porcar, E., Pons, A.M. & Lorente, A. Visual and ocular effects from the use of flat-panel displays, *Int J Ophthalmol* 2016, 9(6): 881-5

Shantakumari, N., Eldeeb, R., Sreedharan, J. & Gopal, K. Computer use and vision-related problems among university students in Ajman, United Arab Emirate. *Ann Med Health Sci Res* 2014, 4(2):258-63

Montagni I, Guichard E, Carpenet C, Tzourio C, Kurth T. Screen time exposure and reporting of headaches in young adults: A cross-sectional study. *Cephalalgia* 2015, Dec 2

Malkki H. Migraine: Long screen time exposure could increase the risk of migraine. *Nature Reviews Neurology* 2015, Dec 18;12(1)

1.10 Loneliness and isolation

Holt-Lunstad J, Smith TB, Layton JB. Social relationships and mortality risk: A meta-analytic review. *PLOS Med 2010*, Jul 27;7(7):e1000316

Gerst-Emerson K, Jayawardhana J. Loneliness as a public health issue: The impact of loneliness on health care utilization among older adults. *Am J Public Health* 2015, May;105(5):1013-9

Holt-Lunstad J, Smith TB, Baker M, Harris T, Stephenson D. Loneliness and social isolation as risk factors for mortality: A meta-analytic review. *Perspect Psychol Sci* 2015, Mar;10(2):227-37

Belojevic G, Slepcevic V, JakovljevicC B. Mental performance in noise: The role of introversion. *Journal of Environmental Psychology* 2001, Jun;21(2):209-13

Shettar M, Karkal R, Kakunje A, Mendonsa RD, Chandran VM. Facebook addiction and loneliness in the postgraduate students of a university in southern India. *Int J Soc Psychiatry* 2017, Jun;63(4):325-9

1.11 Weight gain and weight loss

Caballero B. The global epidemic of obesity: An overview. *Epidemiologic Reviews* 2007, Jan;29(1):1-5

Swinburn BA, Sacks G, Hall KD, et al. The global obesity pandemic: shaped by global drivers and local environments. *Lancet* 2011, Aug 27;378(9793):804-14

Royal Society for Public Health. *Size Matters: The impact of upselling on weight gain.* London: 2017

Centers for Disease Control and Prevention. Further information on diabetes prevalence in the USA. https://www.cdc.gov/diabetes/basics/diabetes.html

1.14 Digestive issues and IBS

Nanayakkara WS, Skidmore PM, O'Brien L, Wilkinson TJ, and Gearry RB. Efficacy of the low FODMAP diet for treating irritable bowel syndrome: the evidence to date. Clin Exp Gastroenterol. New Zealand; 2016;9:131-42

Zhang Y, Li L, Guo C, et al. *BMC Gastroenterol* 2016 June 13;16(1);62. Effects of probiotic type, dose and treatment duration on irritable bowel syndrome diagnosed by Rome III criteria: a meta-analysis

Kings College London information on the low FODMAP diet. https://www.kcl.ac.uk/lsm/research/divisions/dns/projects/fodmaps/faq.aspx

Monash University FODMAP https://www.monashfodmap.com/

1.15 Mood and mental health

Stathopoulou G, Powers MB, Berry AC, Smits JAJ, Otto MW. Exercise interventions for mental health: A quantitative and qualitative review. *Clinical Psychology: Science and Practice* 2006, May;13(2):179-93

Bize R, Johnson JA, Plotnikoff RC. Physical activity level and health-related quality of life in the general adult population: A systematic review. *Prev Med* 2007, Dec;45(6):401-15

Jayakody K, Gunadasa S, Hosker C. Exercise for anxiety disorders: Systematic review. *Br J Sports Med* 2014, Feb;48(3):187-96

Herring MP, Jacob ML, Suveg C, Dishman RK, O'Connor PJ. Feasibility of exercise training for the short-term treatment of generalized anxiety disorder: A randomized controlled trial. *Psychother Psychosom* 2012;81(1):21-8

Cramer H, Lauche R, Langhorst J, Dobos G. Yoga for depression: a systematic review and meta-analysis. *Depression and Anxiety* 2013, Nov;30(11):1068-83

Cramer H, Anheyer D, Lauche R, Dobos G. A systematic review of yoga for major depressive disorder. *J Affect Disord* 2017, Apr 15;213:70-7

1.18 Alcohol

Ludwig AM. Alcohol input and creative output. *Br J Addict* 1990, Jul;85(7):953-63

Lapp WM, Collins RL, Izzo CV. On the enhancement of creativity by alcohol: Pharmacology or expectation? *Am J Psychol* 1994;107(2):173-206

Jarosz AF, Colflesh GJ, Wiley J. Uncorking the muse: Alcohol intoxication facilitates creative problem solving. *Conscious Cogn* 2012, Mar;21(1):487-93

1.19 Coffee

Gunter MJ, Murphy N, Cross AJ, Dossus L, Dartois L, Fagherazzi G, et al. Coffee drinking and mortality in 10 European countries: A multinational cohort study. *Ann Intern Med* 2017, Jul 11

Shammas MA. Telomeres, lifestyle, cancer, and aging. *Curr Opin Clin Nutr Metab Care* 2011, Jan;14(1):28-34

Wikoff D, Welsh BT, Henderson R, Brorby GP, Britt J, Myers E, et al. Systematic review of the potential adverse effects of caffeine consumption in healthy adults, pregnant women, adolescents, and children. *Food Chem Toxicol* 2017, Apr 21

Caini S, Masala G, Saieva C, Kvaskoff M, Savoye I, Sacerdote C, et al. Coffee, tea and melanoma risk: Findings from the European prospective investigation into cancer and nutrition. *Int J Cancer* 2017, May 15;140(10):2246-55

Addicott MA. Caffeine use disorder: A review of the evidence and future implications. *Curr Addict Rep* 2014, Sep;1(3):186-92

1.20 Supplements, substances and nootropics

Radhakrishnan R, Wilkinson ST, D'Souza DC. Gone to Pot - A review of the association between cannabis and psychosis. *Front Psychiatry.* 2014 May 22;5:54

Effects of cannabis use on human behavior, including cognition, motivation, and psychosis: a review. *JAMA Psychiatry* 2016;73:292-7

Battleday RM, Brem A-K. Modafinil for cognitive neuroenhancement in healthy non-sleep-deprived subjects: A systematic review. *Eur Neuropsychopharmacol* 2015;25:1865-81

2.1 Improve your work place

Jacobs K, Foley G, Punnett L, Hall V, Gore R, Brownson E, et al. University students' notebook computer use: Lessons learned using e-diaries to report musculoskeletal discomfort. *Ergonomics* 2011, Feb;54(2):206-19

Shrestha N, Kukkonen-Harjula KT, Verbeek JH, Ijaz S, Hermans V, and Bhaumik S. Workplace interventions for reducing sitting at work. *Cochrane Database Syst Rev.* England; 2016;3:CD010912

MacEwen BT, MacDonald DJ, and Burr JF. A systematic review of standing and treadmill desks in the workplace. *Prev Med.* United States; 2015;70:50-8

Larson MJ, LeCheminant JD, Hill K, Carbine K, Masterson T, and Christenson E. Cognitive and typing outcomes measured simultaneously with slow treadmill walking or sitting: implications for treadmill desks. *PLOS One.* United States; 2015;10(4):e0121309

2.2 Sort out your sleep

Falloon K, Arroll B, Elley CR, et al; The assessment and management of insomnia in primary care. *BMJ.* 2011 May 27 342:d2899

Meolie AL, Rosen C, Kristo D, Kohrman M, Gooneratne N, Aguillard RN, et al. Oral nonprescription treatment for insomnia: An evaluation of products with limited evidence. *J Clin Sleep Med* 2005, Apr 15;1(2):173-87

Rondanelli M, Opizzi A, Monteferrario F, Antoniello N, Manni R, Klersy C. The effect of melatonin, magnesium, and zinc on primary insomnia in long-term care facility residents in italy: A double-blind, placebo-controlled clinical trial. *J Am Geriatr Soc* 2011, Jan;59(1):82-90

Abbasi B, Kimiagar M, Sadeghniiat K, Shirazi MM, Hedayati M, Rashidkhani B. The effect of magnesium supplementation on primary insomnia in elderly: A double-blind placebo-controlled clinical trial. *J Res Med Sci* 2012, Dec;17(12):1161-9

Park CH, Kim EH, Roh YH, Kim HY, Lee SK. The association between the use of proton pump inhibitors and the risk of hypomagnesemia: A systematic review and meta-analysis. *PLOS One* 2014;9(11):e112558

Seyffert M, Lagisetty P, Landgraf J, Chopra V, Pfeiffer PN, Conte ML, Rogers MA. Internet-Delivered cognitive behavioral therapy to treat insomnia: A systematic review and meta-analysis. *PLOS One* 2016;11(2):e0149139

Trauer JM, Qian MY, Doyle JS, Rajaratnam SM, Cunnington D. Cognitive behavioral therapy for chronic insomnia: A systematic review and meta-analysis. *Ann Intern Med* 2015, Aug 4;163(3):191-204

Freeman D, Sheaves B, Goodwin GM, Yu L, Nickless A, Harrison PJ, et al. The effects of improving sleep on mental health (OASIS): A randomised controlled trial with mediation analysis. *Lancet Psychiatry* 2017, Oct;4(10):749-758

2.3 Sort out your diet

Dernini S, Berry EM, Serra-Majem L, *et al.* Med Diet 4.0: the Mediterranean diet with four sustainable benefits. *Public Health Nutr* 2017;**20**:1322–30

Martínez-González MA. Benefits of the Mediterranean diet beyond the Mediterranean Sea and beyond food patterns. *BMC Med* 2016;**14**:157

2.5 Sort out your back

Paige NM, Miake-Lye IM, Booth MS, Beroes JM, Mardian AS, Dougherty P, et al. Association of spinal manipulative therapy with clinical benefit and harm for acute low back pain: Systematic review and meta-analysis. *JAMA* 2017, Apr 11;317(14):1451-60

Cramer H, Haller H, Lauche R, Dobos G. Mindfulness-based stress reduction for low back pain. A systematic review. *BMC Complementary and Alternative Medicine* 2012, Sep;12(1):162

Woodman, J.P. & Moore, N.R. Evidence for the effectiveness of Alexander Technique lessons in medical and health-related conditions: a systematic review, *International Journal of Clinical Practice* 2012; 66(1):98-112

Saragiotto BT, Yamato TP, Maher C. Yoga for low back pain: PEDro systematic review update. *Br J Sports Med* 2015, Oct;49(20):1351

Wieland LS, Skoetz N, Pilkington K, Vempati R, D'Adamo CR, Berman BM. Yoga treatment for chronic non-specific low back pain. *Cochrane Database Syst Rev* 2017;1:CD010671

Yamato TP, Maher CG, Saragiotto BT, Hancock MJ, Ostelo RW, Cabral CM, et al. Pilates for low back pain. *Cochrane Database Syst Rev* 2015, Jul 2(7):CD010265

Miyamoto GC, Costa LO, Cabral CM. Efficacy of the pilates method for pain and disability in patients with chronic nonspecific low back pain: A systematic review with meta-analysis. *Braz J Phys Ther* 2013;17(6):517-32

da C Menezes Costa L, Maher CG, Hancock MJ, McAuley JH, Herbert RD, Costa LO. The prognosis of acute and persistent low-back pain: A meta-analysis. *CMAJ* 2012, Aug 7;184(11):E613-24

Wertli MM, Rasmussen-Barr E, Held U, Weiser S, Bachmann LM, Brunner F. Fear-avoidance beliefs-a moderator of treatment efficacy in patients with low back pain: A systematic review. *Spine J* 2014, Nov 1;14(11):2658-78

Smith BE, Littlewood C, May S. An update of stabilisation exercises for low back pain: A systematic review with meta-analysis. *BMC Musculoskelet Disord* 2014, Dec 9;15:416

Cramer H, Lauche R, Haller H, Dobos G. A systematic review and meta-analysis of yoga for low back pain. *Clin J Pain* 2013, May;29(5):450-60

Sitthipornvorakul E, Janwantanakul P, Lohsoonthorn V. The effect of daily walking steps on preventing neck and low back pain in sedentary workers: A 1-year prospective cohort study. *Eur Spine J* 2015, Mar;24(3):417-24

Shiri R, Falah-Hassani K. Does leisure time physical activity protect against low back pain? Systematic review and meta-analysis of 36 prospective cohort studies. *Br J Sports Med* 2017, Jun 14

Wells C, Kolt GS, Marshall P, Hill B, Bialocerkowski A. The effectiveness of pilates exercise in people with chronic low back pain: A systematic review. *PLOS One* 2014;9(7):e100402

Lawford BJ, Walters J, Ferrar K. Does walking improve disability status, function, or quality of life in adults with chronic low back pain? A systematic review. *Clin Rehabil* 2016, Jun;30(6):523-36

Lin CW, McAuley JH, Macedo L, Barnett DC, Smeets RJ, Verbunt JA. Relationship between physical activity and disability in low back pain: A systematic review and meta-analysis. *Pain* 2011, Mar;152(3):607-13

Cramer H, Ward L, Saper R, Fishbein D, Dobos G, Lauche R. The safety of yoga: A systematic review and meta-analysis of randomized controlled trials. *Am J Epidemiol* 2015, Aug 15;182(4):281-93

Enthoven WTM, Roelofs PD, Koes BW. NSAIDs for chronic low back pain. *JAMA* 2017;317(22):2327-8

Deyo RA. The role of spinal manipulation in the treatment of low back pain. *JAMA* 2017;317(14):1418-9

Traeger AC, Hübscher M, Henschke N, Moseley GL, Lee H, McAuley JH. Effect of primary care-based education on reassurance in patients with acute low back pain: Systematic review and meta-analysis. *JAMA Intern Med* 2015, May;175(5):733-43

Posadzki P, Ernst E. Yoga for low back pain: A systematic review of randomized clinical trials. *Clinical Rheumatology* 2011, May;30(9):1257

Balagué F, Mannion AF, Pellisé F, Cedraschi C. Non-specific low back pain. *Lancet* 2012, Feb 4;379(9814):482-91

2.9 Strategies for the sofa-bound

Funk M, Taylor EL. Pedometer-based walking interventions for free-living adults with type 2 diabetes: A systematic review. *Curr Diabetes Rev* 2013, Nov;9(6):462-71

Mansi S, Milosavljevic S, Baxter GD, Tumilty S, Hendrick P. A systematic review of studies using pedometers as an intervention for musculoskeletal diseases. *BMC Musculoskelet Disord* 2014, Jul 10;15:231

Bravata DM, Smith-Spangler C, Sundaram V, Gienger AL, Lin N, Lewis R, et al. Using pedometers to increase physical activity and improve health: A systematic review. *JAMA* 2007, Nov 21;298(19):2296-304

Cayir Y, Aslan SM, Akturk Z. The effect of pedometer use on physical activity and body weight in obese women. *Eur J Sport Sci* 2015;15(4):351-6

Orr K, Howe HS, Omran J, Smith KA, Palmateer TM, Ma AE, Faulkner G. Validity of smartphone pedometer applications. *BMC Res Notes* 2015, Nov 30;8:733

Lauche R, Langhorst J, Lee MS, Dobos G, Cramer H. A systematic review and meta-analysis on the effects of yoga on weight-related outcomes. *Prev Med* 2016;87:213-32

2.15 Build well-being with mindfulness

Tang YY, Lu Q, Geng X, Stein EA, Yang Y, Posner MI. Short-term meditation induces white matter changes in the anterior cingulate. *Proc Natl Acad Sci* USA 2010, Aug 31;107(35):15649-52

Paulson S, Davidson R, Jha A, Kabat-Zinn J. Becoming conscious: The science of mindfulness. *Ann N Y Acad Sci* 2013, Nov;1303:87-104

Tang YY, Hölzel BK, Posner MI. The neuroscience of mindfulness meditation. *Nat Rev Neurosci* 2015, Apr;16(4):213-25

Khoury B, Sharma M, Rush SE, Fournier C. Mindfulness-based stress reduction for healthy individuals: A meta-analysis. *J Psychosom Res* 2015, Jun;78(6):519-28

Cherkin DC, Sherman KJ, Balderson BH, Cook AJ, Anderson ML, Hawkes RJ, et al. Effect of mindfulness-based stress reduction vs cognitive behavioral therapy or usual care on back pain and functional limitations in adults with chronic low back pain: A randomized clinical trial. *JAMA* 2016;315(12):1240-9

About Joanna Penn

Joanna Penn is a New York Times and USA Today bestselling author of thrillers and dark fantasy under J.F.Penn. She also writes inspirational non-fiction for authors and is an award-winning creative entrepreneur and international professional speaker.

Her site, TheCreativePenn.com is regularly voted one of the top 10 sites for writers and self-publishers. Joanna also has a popular podcast for writers, The Creative Penn.

Joanna has a Master's degree in Theology from the University of Oxford, Mansfield College, and a Graduate Diploma in Psychology from the University of Auckland, New Zealand. She lives in Bath, England but spent 11 years living in Australia and New Zealand. Joanna enjoys traveling as often as possible. She's interested in religion and psychology and loves to read, drink gin and tonic, and soak up European culture through art, architecture and food.

Connect with Joanna online:

www.TheCreativePenn.com/contact
Twitter.com/thecreativepenn
Facebook.com/TheCreativePenn
Youtube.com/thecreativepenn

Joanna also has a popular podcast for writers,
TheCreativePenn.com/podcasts/

Joanna's fiction site: www.JFPenn.com

Other Books by Joanna Penn

Get your FREE Successful Author Blueprint
and video series:

www.TheCreativePenn.com/blueprint

More Books for Writers

How to Make a Living with Your Writing:
Books, Blogging and More

Successful Self-Publishing:
How to publish an ebook and a print book

How to Market a Book Third Edition

The Successful Author Mindset

Public Speaking for Authors,
Creatives, and Other Introverts

Co-Writing a Book: Collaboration and
Co-creation for Writers

Business for Authors: How to be an Author Entrepreneur

Career Change: Stop Hating your Job, Discover
What you Really Want to Do, and Start Doing It

* * *

Thrillers by J.F.PENN

Get a free thriller: www.JFPenn.com/free

ARKANE Thrillers

Stone of Fire #1
Crypt of Bone #2
Ark of Blood #3
One Day in Budapest #4
Day of the Vikings #5
Gates of Hell #6
One Day in New York #7
Destroyer of Worlds #8
End of Days #9

London Crime Thrillers

Desecration #1
Delirium #2
Deviance #3

Mapwalker Dark Fantasy series

Map of Shadows #1

Standalone Fantasy Thrillers

Risen Gods - with J.Thorn

A Thousand Fiendish Angels

American Demon Hunters: Sacrifice
- with J. Thorn, Lindsay Buroker, Zach Bohannon

About Euan Lawson

Euan Lawson is an ex-British Army doctor and a Fellow of the Royal College of General Practitioners. He has a special interest in the management of addictions and he writes regularly on healthy habits.

Euan lives in Cumbria, England with his wife and three children. He was into mountaineering and ice climbing in his younger days but he now prefers to get his fix of the outdoors by running across the fells with his sprocker spaniel, Minnie. He also writes fiction and reviews at the website Crime Fiction Lover.

While he can run up a hill or two and enjoy a triathlon, he is contentedly resigned to the fact that the words chiseled and buff will never be used to describe him. He still eats too many crisps.

Not everything in life can be subjected to a randomized controlled trial but he likes to take an evidence-based approach to health. He is keen to help normal men get a little fitter and live a happier, healthier life.

Get your FREE Healthy Bloke Action Plan:

www.euanlawson.com/healthybloke

Connect with Euan:

www.euanlawson.com
euan@euanlawson.com
Twitter.com/euan_lawson

Acknowledgments

Thanks to Dan Holloway, performance poet and author, for the chapter on Riding the Waves.

Thanks to Jonathan for sharing his personal journey of IBS and FODMAP.

Thanks to Simona Hernandez at Yoga Bodhi, Bath, whose expert teaching and gentle joy have transformed my back pain and given me a sustaining yoga practice.

Thanks to everyone who completed The Healthy Writer Survey on The Creative Penn in 2017. Special thanks to those quoted in the book:

AJ, Alexa, Becky, CM Barrett, Shelley Sperry, Lynn Cahoon, Halona Black, Christa Geraghty, Lydiae, EM Atkinson, John Lilley, Maryann Jacobsen, Clare Lydon, Tracy Line, Steven Turner, Nicole Evelina, Jamee Thumm, Robin C Farrell, Stephanie Cain, Christine J Laurenson, Andrew Turpin, Joe Baird, Jade Campbell, Abigail Dunard, Michelle Laurie, Lesley Galston, Gabrielle Garbin, Sandy Vaile, Traveller, Ethan Freckleton, Carrie McAllister, Steven Hayward, Janine Senyszyn, Rhonda, Mark Dawson, Imogen Clark, Louise Waghorn, Marianne Sciucco, Dr Pranathi Kondapaneni, Leah Cutter, Kristine Kathryn Rusch, Jan Hawke, Angela Clarke, Rebecca Bradley.

Thanks to Jane Dixon Smith at JD Smith Design for the book cover and interior print design, to Liz Dexter for proofreading, and to Alexandra Amor for beta reading and double-checking attributions.

Lightning Source UK Ltd.
Milton Keynes UK
UKHW02f1000131217
314388UK00006B/104/P